THE
L·O·N·G·E·VI·T·Y
PROJECT

THE L·O·N·G·E·V·I·T·Y PROJECT

Surprising Discoveries for Health and Long Life from the Landmark Eight-Decade Study

Howard S. Friedman, Ph.D.,
and Leslie R. Martin, Ph.D.

HUDSON
STREET
PRESS

HUDSON STREET PRESS
Published by Penguin Group
Penguin Group (USA) Inc., 375 Hudson Street, New York, New York 10014, U.S.A. • Penguin Group (Canada), 90 Eglinton Avenue East, Suite 700, Toronto, Ontario, Canada M4P 2Y3 (a division of Pearson Penguin Canada Inc.) • Penguin Books Ltd, 80 Strand, London WC2R oRL, England • Penguin Ireland, 25 St Stephen's Green, Dublin 2, Ireland (a division of Penguin Books Ltd) • Penguin Group (Australia), 250 Camberwell Road, Camberwell, Victoria 3124, Australia (a division of Pearson Australia Group Pty Ltd) • Penguin Books India Pvt Ltd, 11 Community Centre, Panchsheel Park, New Delhi – 110 017, India • Penguin Group (NZ), 67 Apollo Drive, Rosedale, North Shore 0632, New Zealand (a division of Pearson New Zealand Ltd) • Penguin Books (South Africa) (Pty) Ltd, 24 Sturdee Avenue, Rosebank, Johannesburg 2196, South Africa

Penguin Books Ltd, Registered Offices: 80 Strand, London WC2R 0RL, England

First published by Hudson Street Press, a member of Penguin Group (USA) Inc.

First Printing, March 2011
10 9 8 7 6 5 4 3 2 1

REGISTERED TRADEMARK—MARCA REGISTRADA
HUDSON
STREET
PRESS

LIBRARY OF CONGRESS CATALOGING-IN-PUBLICATION DATA
Friedman, Howard S.
  The longevity project : surprising discoveries for health and long life from the landmark eight-decade study / Howard S. Friedman and Leslie R. Martin.
    p. cm.
  Includes index.
  ISBN 978-1-59463-075-0
1. Longevity. I. Martin, Leslie R. II. Title.
  RA776.75.F75 2010
  613.2—dc22

Printed in the United States of America
Set in Warnock Pro • Designed by Eve L. Kirch

PUBLISHER'S NOTE
Every effort has been made to ensure that the information contained in this book is complete and accurate. However, neither the publisher nor the author is engaged in rendering professional advice or services to the individual reader. The ideas, procedures, and suggestions contained in this book are not intended as a substitute for consulting with your physician. All matters regarding your health require medical supervision. Neither the author nor the publisher shall be liable or responsible for any loss or damage allegedly arising from any information or suggestion in this book

BOOKS ARE AVAILABLE AT QUANTITY DISCOUNTS WHEN USED TO PROMOTE PRODUCTS OR SERVICES FOR INFORMATION PLEASE WRITE TO PREMIUM MARKETING DIVISION, PENGUIN GROUP (USA) INC., 375 HUDSON STREET, NEW YORK, NEW YORK 10014.

To Dr. Terman, the Terman participants,
and our many fellow Termanators

· CONTENTS ·

viii   Contents

· INTRODUCTION ·

The Breakthrough Studies of a Lifetime

In September 1921, a talented young schoolgirl named Patricia and her precocious classmate John were pulled out of their San Francisco classrooms by a Stanford University psychologist, Lewis Terman. Dr. Terman was looking for gifted children and had asked their teachers to pick out the brightest kids in the class. He was interested in the sources of intellectual leadership and wondered if he could identify early glimmers of high potential.

Eighty years later, both Patricia and John were still alive at ninety-one years old. They had beaten the odds and lived very long and healthy lives. What was their secret? In an effort to find out, we have spent the past twenty years following up on the people in Dr. Terman's studies and investigating why some people thrive well into old age while others fall ill and die prematurely. Along the way, we've discovered that many common health recommendations are ill-advised or simply wrong. We've replaced those with more accurate guideposts to a longer, healthier life.

The 1,500 or so bright boys and girls selected by Dr. Terman were born around 1910. Almost all of them are now gone. We have documented when and how they died, and we have studied their lives in meticulous detail. Although many died by their sixties, many others aged in good health and lived well into old age. Surprisingly, the long-lived among them did not find the secret to health in broccoli, medical tests, vitamins, or jogging. Rather, they were individuals with certain constellations of habits and patterns of living. Their personalities, career trajectories, and social lives proved highly relevant to their long-term health, often in ways we did not expect.

The usual piecemeal suggestions given to those who want to improve their health ("relax," "eat vegetables," "lose weight," "get married") are lifesaving for some but neither effective nor economical for many. In fact, standard medical advice often backfires, leaving us overweight and overstressed as we struggle to follow specific edicts. Our society spends a fortune on health care, fad diets, pharmaceuticals, and a variety of short-term remedies that help somewhat; but there is often disappointingly little effect on our long-term health and longevity.

The late comedian and actress Lucille Ball had her own secret to staying young: live honestly, eat slowly, and lie about your age.[1] Lucy was both right and wrong. Living honestly, our data show, really can be important, but eating slowly doesn't much matter. Lying about your age and your health does indeed represent a challenge to health researchers, but we have figured out ways to outwit the Lucys of the world and get around this common source of research bias.

In our studies we focus first on longevity—length of life. Many studies of well-being are flawed because they rely too heavily on participants' answers to queries about their health and wellness—called their "self-report." Their self-reported answers are subjective and often inaccurate. Longevity is not distorted by self-report. Although there is a field of study on the reliability of death certificates, it is pretty much the case that if your death certificate says that you died on April 26, 1989, then we can be reasonably certain of your longevity and of your state of health on that date. Lucille Ball was not a participant in Dr. Terman's studies, but, as we shall see, one of her closest associates was.

Many common beliefs about health and longevity come from a host of biased sources—with distortions that go well beyond the self-report biases. Aside from the self-interest research biases we hear so much about (in which someone has a financial stake in the findings), there are also many sources of inadvertent skew or error. If you think about it—as we do every day in our laboratory—you come to realize that we can never be quite sure about the validity of many health studies and claims.

Of course we can study individuals who stay healthy, but to whom do we compare them? If we knew that two people started out exactly the same at birth but one ate only broccoli while the other ate only fried steak, then we might have a reasonable comparison. But almost all epidemiological studies, even those making daily headlines, compare people who differ in many, many ways. Indeed they differ in ways we cannot know about. Most comparisons of vegetarians and cheeseburger addicts, or of pill-takers and the pill-averse, therefore are necessarily somewhat flawed. The researchers generally do their best to be as accurate as possible, but there are always limits in a complex study of human health. And the statistics that emerge from the studies can be interpreted in many different ways.

One of the best ways to avoid research traps and biases is to follow individuals for their entire lives and see which characteristics influence subsequent qualities, behaviors, and outcomes. What exactly causes people with similar backgrounds to diverge in terms of their health and well-being? This step-by-step procedure is exactly what we have done, and this book is the first comprehensive report of the findings.

Tracing the lives of hundreds of individuals, we have discovered new twists to common health recommendations, such as when staying single or getting divorced can be healthy for women. Our studies have uncovered a series of what we call dead-end myths—common advice that is not supported by good science and can lead to dead ends in more than one sense of the term. Throughout this book, we'll explain exactly why the following common beliefs, to name a few, are *false*:

The best of men cannot suspend their fate: The good die early, and
   the bad die late. (Myth!)
Get married and you will live longer. (Myth!)

Take it easy and don't work so hard and you will stay healthier. (Myth!)

Thinking happy thoughts reduces stress and leads to long life. (Myth!)

Religious people live longer, so don't miss religious services. (Myth!)

If you have hobbies like gardening, walking, and cooking, you should take up more vigorous forms of exercise. (Myth!)

Worrying is very bad for your health. (Myth!)

If you believe that you are loved and cared for, then you are on the road to good health. (Myth!)

Retire as soon as you can and play more golf to stay healthy and live longer. (Myth!)

If your child is very serious, encourage him or her to be more spontaneous and have more fun. (Myth!)

Give your children a big head start in school and they will thrive for life. (Myth!)

You can live to be a hundred only if you give up all the things that make you want to live to be a hundred (as Woody Allen is said to have joked). (Myth!)

Most books about health and longevity are cookbooks—literally or figuratively. When they aren't giving you recipes (start Week 1 with spinach sautéed in garlic and olive oil) and food lists (an apple a day), they're offering a list of ten dos and don'ts (do exercise for thirty minutes four times a week; don't let your weight rise above a certain ratio to your height).

Exercise, diet, stress, and weight are indeed relevant to health, but in ways that vary from person to person. Lists of dos and don'ts are nearly impossible for most of us to follow for days, months, and years. Thankfully, the Terman study participants showed us that struggling with lists of specific health rules is unnecessary. The Terman men and women were born decades before running shoes, designer spas, and fancy medical tests were invented, yet many lived long, healthy lives. We'll show why.

The point of describing our findings is not to lay out the factors that are likely to leave you the last one standing. Most of us, after all, would not wish to live extra years if they were years of constant decline and pain. But the fact is, those who live longer are also generally healthier throughout their lives. Most people who live to old age do so not because they have beaten cancer, heart disease, diabetes, or lung disease; rather, the long-lived have mostly avoided serious ailments altogether.

Because Dr. Terman began studying his participants when they were very young, many of the insights that emerged are helpful not only to adults looking to get on a healthier life path but also to those hoping to set their children on a good track. Many of our findings can help people rethink the potential long-term effects of their parenting decisions, as well as promote their whole family's future health, happiness, and well-being.

We found that those who are healthier tend to be happier, and those who are happier tend to be healthier—but not for the reasons you might first imagine! The lives of the Terman participants open a new window to understanding the intriguing relationship between health and happiness. Our research yielded powerful suggestions for cultivating not only a long life but also a successful, meaningful, and productive life.

The Amazing Study

When Dr. Terman began studying Patricia and John and these hundreds of other bright boys and girls in California, he collected all sorts of valuable information about the children's families, schooling, and activities. He recorded how many books were in their houses, how active they were in their playtime, and how happy their parents' marriages were. He measured their personalities—were they prudent, extroverted, cheerful? He then followed his participants as they grew up, made career choices, and had families of their own.

When he launched the study in 1921, Dr. Terman was in his mid-forties. He died in 1956, but the project continued, carried on by others. We began serious work on this study in 1990 and so often use the phrases "our study" or "our project" when talking about analyses, findings, and interpretations. But this is not in any way intended to ignore or minimize the tremendous debt we all owe to Dr. Terman, to his collaborators, and to the Terman participants and their families.

A key to success for much of our work on better understanding health and longevity was gathering the death certificates of Terman's study participants from states and counties across the United States. It turned out to be a very difficult and time-consuming task, as each state, county, or city agency has its own procedures and requirements for obtaining a vital-statistic document like a death certificate. (Here's a tip: if you want to be studied by health researchers, don't die in New York City.) But we persisted and now have this invaluable resource.

Having determined how long each of the Terman participants lived (and the precise cause of death), we were able to design and conduct a series of studies that were never before possible. We used both sophisticated statistical models and a variety of examinations of personalities, social relations, and behaviors. We looked at people who shared characteristics—those with similar personalities, say, or a history of divorce—to see whether those traits predicted their health over time. Many of our findings took us by surprise.

You may be wondering if it's fair to generalize from these Terman study participants, who lived in different times and were mostly bright, educated, and middle class. Are the lessons of their lives applicable to people today? It depends on circumstances: a migrant farm worker with little access to education or health care, or a poverty-stricken peasant infected with HIV, has other, more significant threats to his or her health. However, most readers of this book—people who are bright, educated, and interested in health and success—are usually not that different in relevant ways from the Terman participants.

Still, of utmost importance throughout our work has been the effort to confirm that findings from our studies are highly informative for a general understanding of health and longevity. We therefore have spent much time and effort evaluating whether our results are more widely applicable. The answer is yes. We have used a number of scientific techniques to confirm this point. To validate old scales and measures, we conducted comparison studies using contemporary measures from contemporary samples of young people. We have used various statistical tests and adjustments to see if any significant limits would arise from our particular samples of participants. And, before drawing any firm conclusions, we have always compared our findings to what is more broadly known from other research.

As they grew into middle age, the Terman participants were a productive, intelligent segment of twentieth-century middle-class America. They lived through depression, war, and prosperity. They were engineers, businesspeople, housewives, lawyers, administrators, writers, teachers, and all sorts of other blue- and white-collar workers. Most were not particularly notable on a national scale, although you might recognize a few names. None won a Nobel Prize, became a national political leader, or joined the superrich, although some were very prominent in their fields of endeavor. Some died young and some lived to be a hundred.

One of the accomplished individuals in our study was Jess Oppenheimer, who worked with Lucille Ball to create the *I Love Lucy* show. Although the information in the data archives is strictly confidential, some of the Terman participants proudly identified themselves as part of the project. Mr. Oppenheimer was one of the best known.

Oppenheimer was born in San Francisco in 1913 and lived to age seventy-five. He spent most of his adult life in the entertainment business in Los Angeles. In the 1960s, after *I Love Lucy*, Jess worked on the comedy series *Get Smart*. He married, had children, and later wrote about his career. One hint of his broad-ranging intelligence was that he received a patent in the 1950s for his work on a teleprompterlike device, which Lucy used in reading commercials while looking into the camera lens.

The case of Jess Oppenheimer gives a good illustration of the general biographies of the people we have studied. They grew up in California and often remained there. The male participants gravitated toward what they saw as the interesting industries of the twentieth century—education, engineering, broadcasting, law, finance, aviation, and sales. Many were financially successful but many others were not. There were many clerks and some artists, policemen, and technicians. One became a truck driver.

The women, however, were often limited in their early careers by the societal expectations of the 1930s and 1940s. Accordingly, many became housewives, teachers, librarians, or secretaries. But not Shelley Smith. Ms. Smith (Stanford Class of 1936) went to work for *Life* magazine, where she met and married the photographer Carl Mydans. Covering World War II in Asia, she was captured by the Japanese in Manila and spent many months in a prisoner-of-war camp. Yet she lived a long life and died in 2002 at age eighty-six, survived by her husband, a son, a daughter, four grandchildren, and even one great-grandchild.[2]

Jess Oppenheimer and Shelley Smith Mydans, like most of the Terman participants, were interesting people who, when not at work, were involved with family, friends, and hobbies. Most married and stayed married, but a significant number did not. Some were extroverted and others unsociable. Some were impulsive and others prudent. Many of the Terman participants faced significant personal and social difficulties and did not make it into their seventies and eighties. Some of their life paths led to health and long life while others dramatically increased the risks of illness and premature death.

Do You Fit the Bill? Assess Yourself

Always amusing to us is the way that the most objective health scientists become personally caught up in this research. Whenever we present our scientific findings at a research conference, our fellow professionals immediately try to see if they themselves fit the profile of the long-lived. Although the ability to predict health outcomes in any individual case is limited, it is possible to recognize patterns that can lead to meaningful changes. So throughout this book we present relevant measures and risk assessments—self-quizzes, if you will. Often these include some of the same questions Dr. Terman used decades ago. These assessments also serve to provide a deeper understanding of the ideas we're discussing. For example, here is a typical item (from one of the measures):

I am persistent in the accomplishment of my work and ends.
Not true of me   1 2 3 4 5   Very true of me

In later chapters, we present quizzes and measures (and scoring) that you can use to assess yourself:

- Are you conscientious in a health-relevant sense?
- Do you have a sociable personality? And are you a good emotional communicator?
- Are you a moody worrier?
- Are you a gloomy Chicken Little?
- Did your early education predispose you to long life?
- Are you satisfied with your life in a way that impacts your health?
- How physically active are you—on a scientific scale?
- If married, how happy is your marriage?
- How healthy is your job (for you)?
- How do you score on three key measures of social relationships, and especially on the scale most relevant to long life?
- How does your level of religiosity (or lack thereof) impact your health?
- How masculine or feminine are you?
- Are you at risk from health-harming chronic stress?

The "Termanators"

As they grew older, the children in Dr. Terman's study recognized that they were in a special group and in a special study, although no one thought the study would last more than ten or twenty years, much less for eight decades. Giving their identity a special name, they cleverly called themselves "Terman's Termites" or, more simply, "the Termites."

We sometimes use this nickname, "Termites," when referring to the participants in Terman's project. But there are dangers: at one scientific conference, we attempted to present a technical display called "The Longevity of the Termites," but the conference attendees simply ignored us, walking right by our informative exhibit. They evidently assumed that we were entomologists studying wood-eating social insects. Now we are more careful in our terminology.

In any scientific research project, much of the drudgery of data gathering and handling falls to graduate students, who are apprenticed to more established researchers. Our particular project has attracted a number of remarkable graduate student researchers over the years, but after a while they tired of being known as students of "Dr. Friedman's longevity project developing the Terman data." Back in 2005, our graduate students decided that if the participants could be "Termites," then we researchers could be "Termanators." And so they hung a sign outside our lab door: *The Termanator Lab*.

Because we were working at the University of California in Riverside, only about fifty miles east of Hollywood, the name seemed to fit. Despite the nonviolent nature of our work, the plot is the same—to save human lives.

THE
L·O·N·G·E·V·I·T·Y
PROJECT

CHAPTER 1

Personality and Long Life

Who Stays Well?

Patricia and John, two of the Terman participants who lived the longest, led interesting, but not startling, lives.[3] They encountered adventures and surprises but never won a lottery, crashed their cars, or confronted a kidnapper. In this respect, they were quite different from Ann Hodges, an ordinary American who faced an extraordinary event. On November 30, 1954, a meteorite crashed through the roof and injured thirty-one-year-old Ms. Hodges as she lay dozing on her couch in Oak Grove, Alabama.

If a meteor falls out of the sky and strikes you, there is probably little you could have done to prevent it. Some threats are random and unpredictable, at least as far as one can scientifically judge. But many such seemingly chance events are not totally random. Golfers on a Kansas City course who gather under a tree during a storm are more likely to be struck by lightning, for instance, than is a librarian in Los Angeles (where it rarely even thunders).

Surprisingly, the same is true for health. It is not random who will contract the flu or who will recover quickly. Many health threats are not simply due to bad luck. Rather, there are systematic individual differences in susceptibility to injury and disease, who gets sick and who stays well. Some of these are a function of personality—stable individual differences, including associated biological differences. Others are tied to social relations such as marriage, family, friendship, and religious observance. Still others emerge from stressful challenges and the resources one can muster in facing the stress. Most important is our finding that the risk factors and protective shields do not occur in isolation but bunch together in patterns—the healthy or unhealthy life paths or trails that we call pathways. The pathways to long life had unforeseen twists, many of which amazed us.

Individual Pathways

When young Patricia was led out of her classroom to be tested by Dr. Terman, her parents had recently divorced. Although children of divorce face many risks, including health risks (our studies have confirmed this, as we'll show), Patricia was able to avoid them, partly because she later had a good marriage herself. In contrast, her classmate John went against the grain and never married. Yet he, too, lived a long and healthy life. Our studies of personality, marriage, and longevity showed why. Conventional wisdom failed, but a focus on individual pathways yielded insights and understanding—and allowed us to shatter dead-end myths.

It's especially important to be attuned to your own pathway because modern medical professionals will not do it for you. Most physicians, many of whom are highly trained to heal one specific part or system of the body, don't ask about your personality traits, your activity levels as a child, or your family's history of divorce and remarriage. In fact, if you want to understand how you can find your optimal path to health and long life, modern medicine has relatively little to offer. Instead we need to turn to the contemporary fields of health psychology, medical sociology, life-course epidemiology, genetics, and life-span development.

It is from these modern fields that we have drawn the concepts, scientific measures, and statistical analyses needed to understand why some of the Terman participants thrived while others succumbed. We discovered that people spend too much time worrying about rare events like meteor strikes and pay too little attention to their own inclinations, behavioral patterns, and health trajectories.

Backward Thinking?

If a middle-aged man develops heart disease, his cardiologist typically would not delve deeply into whether he had been a prudent child, if he is successful in his career, or if he had been divorced and remarried. Yet personality, family, work, and social relations turn out to join together and be highly relevant to later healthy or unhealthy paths. Ironically, a philosopher from the Middle Ages might have understood individual differences more quickly than modern-day health professionals do. How did this happen?

In the nineteenth century, a young doctor, the Hungarian physician Ignaz Semmelweis, shocked the medical world by arguing that the often-fatal "child-bed fever" of mothers in labor could be prevented if physicians, midwives, and nurses would wash and disinfect their hands and medical utensils. His brilliant insights were initially met with scorn and disbelief by his contemporaries. Dr. Semmelweis was disheartened and suffered a nervous breakdown, but it was not surprising that his hardworking colleagues resisted the notion that they were contributing to their patients' illnesses.

Not long after, however, the French biochemist Louis Pasteur and his associates experimentally proved the existence of infectious microorganisms—germs. Germ control processes and the pasteurization of milk were developed. In the following decades, medical treatment was revolutionized and standardized care introduced. By 1890, surgeons had fully recognized the importance of sterile operating fields and antiseptics. Modern medicine began to flourish, but—here's the rub—the individual became less of a focus. Before that time, explanations of susceptibility to illness came from traditions that focused not on bacterial invaders but on the individual. For example, for generations, clergy had looked at the person to see what sinful behaviors might have brought on illness; it was clear that only some people were prone to disease, and so repentance or exorcism of evil spirits might be the treatment.

In the age-old philosophical establishments, there was likewise a person-centered focus. Are you someone of healthy temperament, optimism, and ruddy complexion? In the Hippocratic tradition, you would be labeled as *sanguine*—a person with a healthy, balanced supply of blood. For nearly two millennia, followers of the ancient physicians Hippocrates and Galen saw four essentials—the so-called bodily humors—as the key to health. Excessive black bile was said to make one *melancholic*—sad, morose; it was believed to cause depression and degenerative diseases or cancer. Yellow bile in excess would make one *choleric*—peevish, angry, bilious; it was said to produce a bitter, angry personality and was associated with feverish diseases. Finally, phlegm was thought to make one *phlegmatic*—sluggish, unemotional, cold, and apathetic; it was associated for example with rheumatism. We have found that these "bodily humors"—although not scientifically valid in the ancient sense—can have valuable counterparts in modern approaches to health, in the form of scientifically derived personality traits. Personality is an excellent predictor of health and longevity, often in counterintuitive ways.

Back to the Beginning

About twenty years ago, the two of us—one a young professor, the other his energetic new graduate student—were growing frustrated with the current state of research about individual differences, stress, health, and longevity. It was clear that some people were more prone to disease, took longer to recover, or died sooner, while others of the same age were able to thrive. All sorts of explanations were being proposed—anxiety, lack of exercise, nerve-racking careers, risk taking, lack of religion, unsociability, disintegrating social groups, pessimism, poverty, poor access to medical care, and type A behavior patterns—the so-called coronary-prone personality of competing hostilely to do too much in too little time. But there was no good way to test these explanations over the long term.

The best study to address such matters would be one that followed a large number of individuals throughout their lives. It would be a study that measured their personalities, their careers, their habits, their stresses, and their health and longevity. Could we do such a study? It would cost many millions of dollars and, most troublingly, we ourselves would be long dead before the results came in (which would not be much fun at all).

Then one day it struck us. Right down the hall from our lab, one of our colleagues, Dr. Carol Tomlinson-Keasey, was studying women's stress, using an old archive at Stanford University. It was the Terman study. We wondered, could this study be adapted to our needs? The bad news was that little health and longevity information was easily available in the archive. The good news was that it was a life-span, decades-long archive, and the possibilities were enormous if we could gather and add all the needed new information.

After discussing the old data with Dr. Tomlinson-Keasey, we decided that yes, we would spend six months to a year examining predictors of health and longevity among the Terman study participants. Two decades later, we are still at it. The deeper we dig into the lives of these people, the more we understand about the pathways to longevity. (And yet, the occasional college student, hearing about our obsession, will properly advise us, "A twenty-year study! Get a life!")

Dr. Terman had begun collecting his information shortly after World War I. Obviously he could not have used the same kinds of measures and assessments that we would select today. But Dr. Terman's approach was amazingly prescient and smart. He gathered all sorts of facts and data that we have been able to convert into modern measures.

Personality Is Not Set in Stone

If it is true, as Wordsworth put it, that "the Child is father of the Man," then childhood characteristics might lead, step by step, to lifelong patterns of health. For example, a sociable child would likely become a sociable adult, and that might be pertinent to good health. Is this the case? Is early personality very relevant to health in later life? Can childhood personality predict longevity decades into the future? Can we change personality and thereby improve health?

In 1922, Dr. Terman surveyed Patricia's parents and teacher. How prudent was twelve-year-old Patricia? How truthful was she? Was she cheerful, with a sense of humor? Did she prefer to play indoors or outdoors? Did she like to go to parties? Dozens of such questions were asked, and the answers were duly recorded. But most of the rating sheets sat gathering dust in the archive, with no one thinking to see whether personality predicted lifelong health and longevity. Then suddenly one day we were in the right place at the right era, with a convergence of several lines of thought.

Because of doubts raised about the stability of personality, researchers have spent the past twenty-five years documenting what the proponents of the Greek humors knew two millennia ago—some people are indeed more agreeable, worrying, careful, sociable, and creative than others.[4] Although there is tremendous variability, there is also a substantial degree of order and constancy. If you return to your high school reunion many years after graduation, the popular and fast-talking extroverts are most likely to have become the successful salespersons and lawyers.

That said, exciting new lines of research within psychology have begun to show how people can change—albeit slowly and with substantial effort. As we will see, consistently placing oneself in groups where one will meet new people can help turn a temperamentally shy person into more of a (mild) social butterfly, for instance. And if we decide that we want to cultivate a trait such as dependability, we can analyze our actions, act "as if" we already possessed those traits, and vigilantly monitor and correct for any slips back to our baseline way of behaving. All of which is to say that if your personality traits don't match those on the pathways to longevity, you can make an effort to expand those needed aspects. The long-lived Terman participants did.

Personality Detectives on the Case

We dug into Terman's archives. Thousands of pieces of information had been collected on each participant for decades. So we started by examining all the items that seemed relevant to personality. Near the outset, in 1922, each participant's parents (usually the mother, or both parents together) and the teacher were asked to rate the child on dozens of trait dimensions. Dr. Terman's interests were wide-ranging—he attempted to measure the intellectual, volitional, moral, emotional, aesthetic, physical, and social functioning of each child!

For example, using a thirteen-point scale, Patricia's mother and her sixth-grade teacher rated her according to the degree to which she appeared to be popular, cheerful, and prudent, among many other traits and dimensions. The picture that emerged was one of a girl who was well liked but not a leader or the most popular student in the class. She enjoyed school and had excellent attendance, and her teacher reported that she seemed particularly drawn to atlases and encyclopedias. Despite being rather bookish, Patricia was not overly shy, and she spent time regularly with several close friends who shared her interests in birds and other wildlife, knitting, and movie stars. Still, as we examined her life over the years, we began referring to her as Prudent Patricia.

Terman's original personality rating scales, now almost a century old, are remarkably modern in their appearance. We could directly analyze them using modern statistics, and so we derived and validated a small number of core personality traits to understand Patricia and her peers. We called one of these "Sociability" and another "Conscientiousness and Social Dependability."

The Sociability index reflects a tendency to prefer being around others. That is, was the child popular, often a leader, fond of being in large groups, and showing a preference for playing with others and being involved in social activities? Patricia was not particularly popular or social and scored about average on this scale. Terman participant James, on the other hand, was a leader and scored high on this index. James tended to think things out for himself, but he was also quite sensitive to the approval of his peers. Charismatic and exceptionally tactful, James successfully garnered the goodwill of his classmates and had many friends—he was a universal favorite at school.

The Conscientiousness scale combined four other characteristics that parents and teachers had rated: how prudent was the child, how conscientious, how truthful, and how free from vanity and egotism? Some people are clearly more conscientious and dependable than others.

We also measured other core personality traits, such as cheerfulness, moodiness, and more—all of which we'll delve into in later chapters.

•   •   •   •   •

After doing years of work on a research project, a moment of truth approaches. In our case, we had painstakingly put together and validated measures of childhood personality, and we had searched high and low for death certificates.

We initially expected that four or five particular traits might be especially relevant. It would make sense if the most sociable children went on to live long lives. After all, scientific studies have firmly established that individuals who are well integrated into communities are generally healthier, as compared to the lonely recluses. We also thought that the cheerful, optimistic children would probably live long lives. The airwaves are full of advice to "cheer up" to stay healthy.

Highly conscientious individuals, we hypothesized, might stay healthier and live longer—perhaps those who were careful and diligent would take better care of themselves. Finally, we had some ideas about individuals who were worriers, got excited, were easily provoked to anger and distress, and so on. We predicted less healthy fates for the moody and troubled. But it did not really matter what we expected; the findings would speak for themselves. We'd quickly discover that our hypotheses—steeped in conventional wisdom from shorter-term studies of personality and health—would only sometimes be right.

· CHAPTER 2 ·

Long Live the Prudent and Persistent

As our graduate students looked over the initial statistical findings on personality and long life, they gasped and laughed as they read the results: "Howard, that sounds like you!" The findings clearly revealed that the best childhood personality predictor of longevity was conscientiousness—the qualities of a prudent, persistent, well-organized person, like a scientist-professor—somewhat obsessive and not at all carefree.

It was not cheerfulness and it was not having a sociable personality that predicted long life across the ensuing many decades. Certain other factors were also relevant, but the prudent, dependable children lived the longest. The strength of this finding was unexpected, but it proved to be a very important and enduring one.

We had worried that perhaps nothing at all would foretell long life. This first finding demonstrated to us that a trait from childhood could be relevant to health many years later. Now we knew that questions Dr. Terman had asked parents and teachers back in 1922 could in fact predict health and longevity many decades into the future. We celebrated and raised our glasses to the Terman subjects, living and departed.

Assess Yourself

As we noted in the introduction, almost everyone seems to want to see where they fit into the long life picture. Do you match the profiles of the long-lived? We need to reiterate that the ability to predict health and longevity in any individual case is imperfect. But individuals often do recognize healthy or unhealthy patterns in themselves, their friends, or their families. To provide a deeper understanding of our ideas and to encourage movement toward healthier pathways, we offer relevant measures and risk assessments.[5]

Let's start with a personality scale that we developed based on both Dr. Terman's questions and scales and our own research, drawing on excellent work done at the Oregon Research Institute by measurement expert Dr. Lew Goldberg, who oversees a personality "collaboratory." Some of the items here are nearly the same as the ones Terman participants used in assessing themselves in young adulthood.

SELF-ASSESSMENT: A KEY PERSONALITY COMPONENT

To assess a core aspect of personality, decide how well each of the following statements describes you. Be honest, thinking about yourself as you usually are, compared to others who are the same sex and about the same age.

1. I am always prepared.

1 – very inaccurate
2 – moderately inaccurate
3 – neither accurate nor inaccurate
4 – moderately accurate
5 – very accurate

2. I leave my belongings around.

1 – very inaccurate
2 – moderately inaccurate
3 – neither accurate nor inaccurate
4 – moderately accurate
5 – very accurate

3. I actually get cold when I think of something cold.

1 – very inaccurate
2 – moderately inaccurate
3 – neither accurate nor inaccurate
4 – moderately accurate
5 – very accurate

4. I enjoy planning my work in detail.

1 – very inaccurate
2 – moderately inaccurate
3 – neither accurate nor inaccurate
4 – moderately accurate
5 – very accurate

5. I make a mess of things.

1 – very inaccurate
2 – moderately inaccurate
3 – neither accurate nor inaccurate
4 – moderately accurate
5 – very accurate

6. I get chores done right away.

1 – very inaccurate
2 – moderately inaccurate
3 – neither accurate nor inaccurate
4 – moderately accurate
5 – very accurate

7. I have sometimes had to tell a lie.

1 – very inaccurate
2 – moderately inaccurate
3 – neither accurate nor inaccurate
4 – moderately accurate
5 – very accurate

8. I often forget to put things back in their proper place.

1 – very inaccurate
2 – moderately inaccurate
3 – neither accurate nor inaccurate
4 – moderately accurate
5 – very accurate

9. I like order.

1 – very inaccurate
2 – moderately inaccurate
3 – neither accurate nor inaccurate
4 – moderately accurate
5 – very accurate

10. I shirk my duties.

1 – very inaccurate
2 – moderately inaccurate
3 – neither accurate nor inaccurate
4 – moderately accurate
5 – very accurate

11. I follow a schedule.

1 – very inaccurate
2 – moderately inaccurate
3 – neither accurate nor inaccurate
4 – moderately accurate
5 – very accurate

12. I am persistent in the accomplishment of my work and ends.

1 – very inaccurate
2 – moderately inaccurate
3 – neither accurate nor inaccurate
4 – moderately accurate
5 – very accurate

How to compute the total score:

Each item scores from 1 to 5. But for items 2, 5, 8, and 10, you need to reverse the scores. So if you said that "I leave my belongings around" was "very inaccurate" in describing you (a 1), change your score to its opposite, which is a 5. If you gave yourself a 2 you would change this to a 4 and so on. If you said this was neither accurate nor inaccurate, you would leave your score as it is—a 3.

Then eliminate item 3 and item 7. Item 3 ("I actually get cold when I think of something cold") is an irrelevant filler item. Item 7 is a lie scale, in more than one sense of the term. For the remaining ten items, simply sum your scores.

A total score will fall somewhere between 10 and 50. This scale is a good measure of conscientiousness. Total scores between 10 and 24 indicate very low conscientiousness (the lowest quartile or 25 percent in a recent sample of adults). Scores between 37 and 50 suggest exceptionally high conscientiousness.

Another way to understand your own conscientiousness and to make it a more valid assessment is to get the viewpoint of someone else who knows you well. (Remember that in 1921 and 1922, Dr. Terman didn't ask the children about their personalities. Instead he asked their parents and teachers.) People who know you well are generally good judges of your personality, and sometimes the perspective of someone else can be enlightening, helping us to see ourselves more objectively. So use the same scale, but this time, have a friend rate you.

Conscientious Adults: Then and Now

If our unexpected discovery about childhood conscientiousness and its relevance to long life is not a fluke, then we should also be able to find confirming evidence by studying conscientious adults.

Almost two decades after starting, in the summer of 1940, Dr. Terman approached Patricia and the other members of his select study again. He gave them an extensive new series of tests and measures with such questions as "Are you thrifty and careful about making loans?" and "How persistent are you in the accomplishment of your ends?" From these results we worked for months to construct and validate a new series of personality scales. At times, we also incorporated similar questions that Terman asked the participants in 1950.

Studies of health across the life span face an intriguing dilemma. In order to see whether personality in childhood and young adulthood predicts long life, a result that can't be seen until decades later, we necessarily need to use "old" data. In our case, information from the early and mid-twentieth century is being used to predict longevity into the twenty-first century. But years later, new, improved measures are in vogue, and the dusty old measures and techniques are likely subject to criticism. As Dale Carnegie put it, "Any fool can criticize, condemn and complain, and most fools do."[6]

Short of time travel, how can we be sure that the measures we have from the 1920s, 1940s, and 1950s reflect what we understand about personality today? What at first seemed simple gradually became more and more complex. We decided to administer the Terman questionnaire items to a contemporary sample of people. More than a half century after Dr. Terman measured the personality of Patricia at thirty years old, we recruited a new group of young adults in California and asked them the exact same questions. We also recruited a sample of parents to rate their young children on Terman's scales, just as parents of the Terman participants had done in the 1920s.

We then gave these new participants some modern, well-validated personality tests. Through a series of statistical analyses, we were able to check the old data against new data, thereby creating valid, modern personality measures for Patricia and her associates. It was almost as if we had gone back decades and measured Jess Oppenheimer's personality by finding a modern-day doppelganger. We did this in the technical, statistical way, and then, just to be sure, we examined all the scale items in a rational, commonsense manner. Fortunately, all of the data analyses fit together quite well.[7] Dr. Terman's approach to personality holds up nicely and can help us predict our own futures.

Doing the right statistical analyses in such attempts to predict long life is much more difficult than might be imagined. Long-term longitudinal studies are especially challenging because participants come and go, rejoin or drop out, disappear or are discovered, and live or die. In addressing these and related statistical issues, we were fortunate to have Professor Joseph Schwartz as a key research collaborator. Joe has one of best analytic minds in this field.

Revenge of the Virtuous

Conscientiousness, which was the best predictor of longevity when measured in childhood, also turned out to be the best personality predictor of long life when measured in adulthood. The young adults who were thrifty, persistent, detail oriented, and responsible lived the longest. Patricia was one of these, having told Dr. Terman that she enjoyed "planning [her] work in detail" and tended to "drive [herself] steadily." When asked about how she typically pursued goals, she indicated that she was persistent and that she had "definite purposes." Patricia also reported being "thrifty and careful about making loans" and not at all impulsive. In fact, she had done very well in college and was expecting to have a highly successful career.

By the end of the twentieth century, 70 percent of the Terman men and 51 percent of the Terman women had died. It was the unconscientious among them who had been dying in especially large numbers. This confirmation in adulthood was particularly impressive because personality was being measured differently. Conscientiousness in childhood was measured by parent and teacher ratings. Conscientiousness in adulthood was measured by self-report questionnaires—our analyses of how participants described themselves and their activities. In both cases—childhood and adulthood—conscientiousness was the key personality predictor of long life.[8]

Why Do the Conscientious Stay Healthier and Live Longer?

We thought of three possible reasons for why conscientious individuals tend to stay healthier and live longer. To our great surprise, all three are true. The first reason, perhaps most obvious, is that conscientious people do more things to protect their health and engage in fewer activities that are risky. They are less likely to smoke, drink to excess, abuse drugs, or drive too fast. They are more likely to wear seat belts and follow doctors' orders. They are not necessarily risk averse but they tend to be sensible in evaluating how far to push the envelope.

The second, and least obvious, reason for the health benefits of conscientiousness is that some people are biologically predisposed to be both more conscientious and healthier. Not only do they tend to avoid violent deaths and illnesses linked to smoking and drinking, but conscientious individuals are less prone to a whole host of diseases, not just those caused by dangerous habits. We and others are uncovering this startling finding again and again—conscientious folks are less likely to die from all sorts of causes. While we are not yet sure of the precise physiological reasons, it appears likely that conscientious and unconscientious people have different levels of certain chemicals in their brains, including serotonin. Serotonin is the neurotransmitter targeted by antidepressant drugs like Prozac, Paxil, and Zoloft. Individuals with low levels of serotonin tend to be much more impulsive. Importantly, serotonin is also necessary to regulate many health-relevant processes throughout the body, including how much you eat and how well you sleep.

This is no cause for fatalism, however. Neurotransmitter levels can change over time, and being biologically predisposed toward certain physiological processes is not a death sentence any more than being predisposed to depression means you will absolutely fail to thrive and find satisfaction in life. As we will see, some Terman subjects who started out low on conscientiousness (i.e., who were impetuous and impulsive children) led long and healthy lives.

We've saved the best for last. The most intriguing reason conscientious people live longer is that having a conscientious personality leads you into healthier situations and relationships. In other words, it is not only that conscientious people have better health habits and healthier brains, but also that they find their way to happier marriages, better friendships, and healthier work situations. That's right, conscientious people create healthy, long-life pathways for themselves.

In and Out of Conscientiousness

Some people do change, and they travel down a path that leads them far away from the habits of their youth—for good or for ill. While we found a consistent link between dependable kids and their future adult selves, we also confirmed that human beings can be inconsistent creatures. Some wild frat boys quit drinking the morning after their fortieth birthday. Cautious others abandon their sensible lifestyle in midlife and buy a red sports convertible. How is a change in long-term conscientiousness relevant to health?

We decided (with the advice of Dr. Joe Schwartz) to compare four kinds of people:

- The first is someone like Patricia who was highly conscientious (in the top quartile) in both childhood and adulthood.
- The second is an individual who was conscientious in childhood but turned unconscientious by adulthood.
- The third is someone, such as the tactful and charismatic James, who was decidedly low on this trait as a kid but became one of the most conscientious subjects by the time he reached young adulthood.
- The fourth kind was unconscientious in childhood and remained so in adulthood.

We found that those Terman participants who scored high at both points in time had the lowest risk of dying at any given age. Those who scored low at both points in time had the highest risk of dying. And the others, those who had changed their level of conscientiousness, were in between.

Does It Generalize?

The nineteenth-century Lithuanian scholar Yisroel Lipkin (known as Rav Yisroel Salanter) reportedly said that three things can be learned from a train: (a) if you're late a minute you can miss it, (b) even a tiny move off the tracks causes a catastrophe, and (c) if you travel without a ticket you get punished.[9] We do not have a conscientiousness score for Mr. Lipkin, but staying on track with the proper tickets does seem to be an excellent metaphor for a conscientious lifestyle.

But how can we be sure that conscientiousness is as important to us in the twenty-first century as it was to Dr. Terman's subjects (or to Rabbi Lipkin, for that matter)? Our highly conscientious and talented recent graduate student (and now Ph.D.) Margaret (Peggy) Kern addressed this question. Peggy knew that the past decade had seen a number of researchers following up on our findings and conducting many excellent new studies on personality and health. Why not gather them together and combine the results using the statistical technique called meta-analysis?

Although meta-analysis sounds like a Kantian proposition or a therapy for aging Freudians, it is really a fairly straightforward mathematical tool to combine the results of many studies into a single summary. Peggy computer-searched for all the studies ever published that included a conscientiousness-related trait—prudence, responsibility, self-control, or impulsivity—and a measure of longevity. She found twenty studies, with a total of about nine thousand participants. We combined those studies, and the results clearly confirmed our Terman findings—people ranking higher in conscientiousness were less likely to die at any given age.[10] This held true for young people and it held true for sixty-five- to one-hundred-year-olds.

Personality and Chronic Disease

Conscientiousness predicts long life, but what about its relevance to serious chronic disease? Surely other factors matter quite a bit—would they override the importance of conscientiousness? What about diseases like diabetes, hypertension, stroke, lumbago, depression, and bladder disease? Could prudence possibly be relevant?

We teamed up with Columbia University epidemiologist Renee

Goodwin and looked at a nationally representative sample of thousands of Americans, in order to draw from a large body of evidence in a modern national study. As we now expected, unconscientious people were more likely to suffer from each of these chronic conditions. Individuals who measured low on conscientiousness were not only more likely to be clinically depressed, feel anxious, smoke cigarettes, and have high blood pressure and sciatica, but they were also more likely to have tuberculosis, diabetes, joint problems, and strokes.[11]

Of course, many different things contribute to health and longevity: brushing your teeth and being perennially punctual are not the same as discovering the fountain of youth and drinking its dancing waters of healing. We knew this was not the end of our work on personality and health. We needed to know a great deal more about how conscientiousness combined with other traits and pathways to lead to better health and longer life. The surprising and paradoxical findings about cheerfulness, worrying, sociability, and other characteristics are in the pages ahead.

What It Means for You: Guideposts to Health and Long Life

Are conscientious and dependable people also boring and stale? We have found absolutely no evidence for this stereotype. Potential astronauts and military leaders who are slackers and screwballs are generally not the ones launched into space or put in charge of army commands. The careless and sloppy among us are not the ones usually selected to be judges and surgeons and heads of our most esteemed institutions. Many of the most conscientious Terman subjects led exciting and highly rewarding lives.

Conscientious, dependable people stay healthier and live longer. This is not always the case—there are many exceptions to be found—but conscientiousness is a very good predictor. If you are a conscientious person, the news is good—keep doing what you are already doing. If you are like Patricia, your habits, brain biochemistry, and social environment are likely to work together to decrease your risk of poor health and early death. You're at much lower risk of becoming seriously ill, and you probably already worry enough about health-relevant habits and activities. But large numbers of people are not so conscientious. If this describes you, are you doomed?

No, but you're not likely to change your personality or lifestyle rapidly. It doesn't matter how many New Year's resolutions you make. In fact, rapid and pervasive changes are usually quickly abandoned by anyone undertaking them. Lasting adjustments happen with smaller, but progressive, steps.

People can and do slowly change their patterns and their habits when they seek out situations that promote responsibility. For James, the transition took nearly a decade. In 1922 his conscientiousness score was in the lowest 25 percent of participants. His mother and schoolteacher described him as vain and noted that he lived wholly in the present, seeming never to look very far ahead. He wasn't always reliable or truthful, either, according to these important adults in his life. Smart, like all of the subjects, James finished his freshman year of college at the age of seventeen, but he seemed bored by school and was performing far below his abilities. He took a year off (accomplishing little during that time) but at his family's urging he returned to college and, after switching majors twice, finally graduated with a degree in communications.

When James was assessed in 1936 he was working steadily in public relations and had recently gotten married. We have hints from his family about his characteristics in early adulthood—his mother said he had money worries and his wife described him as a nonconformist, but not as impulsive. By the 1940 assessment, however, his conscientiousness score had moved into the upper 25 percent. He liked his work and was now more detail oriented and persistent and had definite goals. He was still somewhat vain, but James's personality profile as he moved into midlife was much more prudent than it had been in his youth. And he survived to a seasoned old age.

James did not become more conscientious overnight. Based on what our data tell us, it is clear that as James gradually took on the responsibilities of a mature adult, he adopted more and more healthy habits. Yes, he maintained and even increased his physical activity, but that by itself wasn't the key to his longevity. What mattered most was that he entered healthier social environments and relationships, which in turn fostered his health. As we will see in later chapters, his marriage was a good one (his wife agreed), and although his job in public relations wasn't highly technical or exotic, he took pride in doing it very well. As an adult, he described himself as an honest person of high integrity. These new habits and relationships, paralleling his slow alteration in personality, provided a solid foundation for James's health and long life. The next puzzle for us to solve would be why James succeeded in this way while others headed down more destructive paths.

· CHAPTER 3 ·

Friendly and Convivial

Healthy or Trivial?

Americans tend to view sociability and extroversion as desirable qualities—we worry about children who are shy. But being very sociable is not always a good thing. Social ties can cut two ways: sometimes healthy and sometimes harmful. For example, friends, acquaintances, and an extended family can be a lifesaver when facing difficult challenges, but the same folks might be bothersome pests if they are intruding when their help is not appreciated. (The comic George Burns is said to have joked that happiness is having a large, loving, caring, close-knit family . . . in another city.) On the other hand, loneliness and the absence of friends can be stressful and unhealthy—unless you are seeking solitude, calm, and self-reflection.

It seemed reasonable to assume that sociable kids would grow into healthier-than-average adults. Constructed in a similar manner to the Conscientiousness index, we created a Sociability index—a personality measure that combined childhood characteristics involving a tendency to prefer being around others: Was the child popular, a leader, fond of being in large groups? Did he or she show a preference for playing with others and being involved in social activities?

Take Paul, for example. He was a "yes" on all counts. Paul was a well-liked, optimistic, and fashionable fifth grader. Self-confident but also attuned to the opinions of others, he was both energetic and popular. Paul's grades were good but his teacher described him as being "interested more in social activities than lessons." He seemed happiest when working in a group, he loved to joke, and, despite being more selfish than average, he was a favorite among his classmates.

Looking across the decades, we found that the sociable children did *not* live longer. Some, including Paul, died young, while others did live into old age, meaning that on average there was no association between being sociable as a child and having a long life. After pondering the matter for six months, we finally figured out a way to get some insight into this paradox. The double-edged nature of sociability helped explain our surprising finding.

The Scientist-Businessman Continuum

In 1954, in one of the last studies he carried out before he died, Dr. Terman posed the question "Are scientists different?" He was wondering how to recruit more scholars to be scientists and also how to smooth relations between scientists and lawyers. (Not long after, the physicist and novelist C. P. Snow famously called the culture gap between scientists and humanists a gulf of mutual incomprehension.)

Dr. Terman, ever the empiricist, looked for the qualities that distinguished subjects who had become scientists from those who had become businessmen, lawyers, and managers. The differences were so vast that he concluded that scientists and engineers are at the *opposite pole* from businessmen and lawyers in their abilities, occupational interests, and social behaviors.

In particular, the scientists were much more unsociable. When they were in school, these future scientists were shyer and less involved in social activities, and when they were young adults, they were less interested in social networks. These differences were just what we needed—an important clue as to why sociability did not predict who lived a long life.

We re-created Dr. Terman's groups of scientists and nonscientists and analyzed how long they lived. The scientists outlived the nonscientists. Only two-thirds of nonscientists but almost three-quarters of scientists lived to reach age seventy.[12]

John was a shy child who tried to avoid playing in large groups; he preferred chess and checkers to tag or charades. He later became a physicist. It was a common pattern: the Terman participants who would go on to be scientists were much less sociable than those who became lawyers, businessmen, and salesmen. The two groups were about equal on the trait of conscientiousness. Dr. Terman asserted that there was no doubt that nonscientists scored higher than scientists in social relations. (In his report, Dr. Terman bragged that he was using the newly developed IBM electrical computers—among the first computers ever used in social science research, and a great aid to statistical computations.)

So why didn't sociability necessarily set one on a path to long life? After all, the sociable children grew up to be adults who had better social relations, and good social relations are normally a sign of good health.

It turns out the scientists had an ace in the hole: they tended to move into stable jobs, have long-lasting marriages, and generally work in a responsible manner. The nonscientists—that is, the businessmen, lawyers, salesmen, and so on—tended to have more tumultuous, less stable, and more health-damaging careers and behaviors. Overall, sociability was a wash. It didn't help or harm one's expected life span. The finding is an excellent reminder that supposed health benefits are often not what they first appear to be. To truly understand them, we have to examine real lives in real contexts, over time.

Sociability and Specific Behaviors

Which aspects of early individual personality characteristics were able to predict unhealthy behaviors in adulthood? Our full team, led by Joan Tucker, a graduate student at the time, identified health-relevant behaviors at midlife, when the Terman participants were about forty to fifty years old. The sociable children grew up to drink more and smoke more over the decades. Unlike the conscientious children, who grew up to behave in healthier ways, people who were more outgoing and sociable were more likely to go along with social pressures toward drinking and smoking.[13] They also more frequently found themselves in an atmosphere where such activities were the "thing to do." Interestingly, there is also substantial scientific evidence (from various investigators) that outgoing, extroverted people find the rewards of an alcohol- or tobacco-induced buzz inherently more appealing.[14]

It was especially intriguing to see that the effects of sociability on health-relevant behaviors held not only in adolescence but also for decades into adulthood.

SELF-ASSESSMENT: SOCIABILITY

For each of the items listed below, choose the response that best represents your feeling.

Fondness for large groups
1 - I love large groups; I am unhappy when alone.
2 - I consider myself to be a "social person."
3 - I consider myself to be something of a "loner."
4 - I always prefer to be alone or with just one or two close friends; I avoid crowds.

Popularity
1 - I have few friends; I am socially shunned.
2 - I'm less popular than average.
3 - I'm pretty popular.
4 - I am well liked; people seek me out and I have many friends.

Spending leisure time

1 - If I had three hours to spend I'd like to attend a party.
2 - If I had three hours to spend I'd want to hang out with a few friends.
3 - If I had three hours to spend I might like to do something with a friend, or maybe not.
4 - If I had three hours to spend I'd relish my solitude and want to spend it doing something by myself.

Life of the party

1 - If a gathering is dull you can bet I won't be doing anything to liven it up.
2 - If a gathering needs livening up, I occasionally try to get it going.
3 - If a gathering is dull I am likely to try to liven it up.
4 - A gathering is never boring when I'm around—I can always keep things exciting.

How to score: For the first and third items, reverse your score (if you said that you love large groups and are unhappy when alone, give yourself a 4, not a 1; or switch a 2 for a 3). Once you've done the reversal, add up your total for all four items; the score should fall between 4 and 16. Paul and his sociable counterparts scored in the double digits, while the more reserved Terman participants like John scored closer to the low of 4. Sociability is one of the personality characteristics that is relatively easy to judge accurately, so you are likely not surprised by your score. We also tend to be good at rating people we meet on this dimension. Because it involves behaviors and characteristics we can readily observe, we quickly get a good sense of who are the popular principals in a group.

As noted, level of sociability is not related to health and longevity in a simple way. As with the scientists, lawyers, and businessmen in Terman's studies, to understand sociability's likely impact, you also need to take into account whether or not your sociability leads you into unhealthy friendships and activities.

Another Kind of Sociability

To delve deeper, we have been studying a special aspect of sociability—
the type of sociability that allows a person to connect emotionally with
others in a powerful way.

SELF-ASSESSMENT: EMOTIONAL SOCIABILITY

*The novel approach we have developed for these issues of emotional
sociability is illustrated by the following scale.*

Not at all true of me   1 2 3 4 5 6 7 8 9   Very true of me

1. When I hear excellent dance music, my
   body immediately starts moving.   1 2 3 4 5 6 7 8 9

2. When I laugh, people know it—it's a hearty
   laugh.   1 2 3 4 5 6 7 8 9

3. I pay attention to details.   1 2 3 4 5 6 7 8 9

4. When I talk on the telephone, my feelings
   and emotions come through loud and clear. 1 2 3 4 5 6 7 8 9

5. I am always prepared.   1 2 3 4 5 6 7 8 9

6. Friends often come to me to tell me their
   problems and seek my advice.   1 2 3 4 5 6 7 8 9

7. I follow a schedule.   1 2 3 4 5 6 7 8 9

8. I continue until everything is perfect.   1 2 3 4 5 6 7 8 9

9. Friends tell me that I should be an actor.   1 2 3 4 5 6 7 8 9

10. I make plans and stick to them.   1 2 3 4 5 6 7 8 9

11. I sometimes forget to put things back in
    their proper place.   1 2 3 4 5 6 7 8 9

12. I am excellent in games like charades,
    where performance and communication
    are important.   1 2 3 4 5 6 7 8 9

13. I am often mistaken for being younger than
    my age.   1 2 3 4 5 6 7 8 9

14. At meetings, barbecues, and other
    gatherings, I am often the center of
    attention.   1 2 3 4 5 6 7 8 9

15. In conversations with people I like, I often
    demonstrate my affection by hugging or
    touching them.   1 2 3 4 5 6 7 8 9

To compute your total score, add the numbers you chose for items 1, 2, 4, 6, 9, 12, 14, and 15. (Disregard the other questions.) Your score should be between 8 and 72. An average score is in the 40s. A score below 36 puts you in the bottom 25 percent. A score above 50 puts you in the upper 25 percent, and a score above 58 is in the top 5 percent.

This latter scale is one of our measures of affective (emotionally motivated) communication—how well one sends his or her feelings to others. People high on this dimension are usually excellent in sales and persuasion. Many of the Terman subjects with these characteristics went on to be leaders in their fields. Because of their enthusiasm, emotional connectedness, and social skills, individuals scoring high on this dimension have an inherent tendency to be healthy, but here again, it can lead to substantial trouble and unhealthy behavior if they are charming their way into risky situations or overindulgent crowds of hedonistic friends. Nevertheless, many individuals strong on affective communication have the emotional skills to allow them to enter very healthy long-term paths, if they choose wisely.

Why Ask Who Lives Longest

Although our studies look at health, aging, happiness, and other signs of well-being, we always ask who lives longest. Why? We start with analyses of longevity because length of life is the single best measure of health. When public health agencies want to assess the overall health of a given country or state, they always start with average life expectancy—for good reason. There are lots of arguments about how to measure quality of life and wellness, but if you are dead, we can be quite sure that you have an extremely low quality of life. And, as noted, if you are on a path to a very long life, you are usually living a very healthy life.

We also wanted full details about *causes* of death—accidents, cancer, heart disease, and so on. So after we painstakingly obtained from state bureaus the death certificates for all the deceased participants, a certified nosologist—a specialist in classifying disease—coded them for underlying cause of death. Dr. Michael Criqui, an expert on cause of death and a physician-epidemiologist, was a key contributor, who also brought an emphasis on healthy behaviors to our studies. Whereas most research on personality and health had previously focused on stress and internal psychological conflict, Mike kept turning our attention back to patterns of healthy and unhealthy behaviors; it was such patterns across time that ultimately proved essential to understanding long life.

What It Means for You: Guideposts to Health and Long Life

The surprising news here is that sociability, generally speaking, isn't as health protective as people think. For parents of shy children or for adults who have always worried whether they should get out and be more interactive, this is good news. Being a "people person" can have its benefits, but those who rank high on sociability often find themselves in environments that encourage unhealthy behaviors—and they join in the dangers of the moment.

To enjoy the perks of a sociable nature while minimizing the risks, our studies suggest being selective about whom you socialize with. As we will see in some detail, those study participants who chose wisely reaped long-term health benefits. Further, many of the more introverted children in our study grew up to take on stable jobs and develop steady friendships, which were just as valuable for health and long life. So if you're socially reluctant and you're okay with that—so are we.

What if you *want* to become less shy and build up a network of healthy friends? Assess yourself on our scale of affective communication, and then approach this challenge by going out and talking to one more additional person each week, paying special attention to the emotional signals you send to others. Looking back over the statements in the second (emotional sociability) self-assessment above, you will see that they hit on nonverbal communication—physical touch, body movement, and expression of feeling through one's voice. Incorporating these elements is important—consider the different reactions you might get when you go out to socialize but you do not communicate emotionally (e.g., by sitting stiffly, making little eye contact, speaking in a monotone) versus when you do communicate well (e.g., by sitting with a relaxed posture, making eye contact, speaking with varying inflections that convey your interest in a subject, showing interest by nodding, and so on). The positive responses you are likely to receive will encourage you to persist in your efforts—our studies show that you will definitely get better with practice, even after a rough start. Socializing is only half the battle; being the type of person that someone else wants to socialize with is the other half.

While sociability by itself turned out not to be the reason some lived longer and others died sooner, this does not mean that social relations are unimportant to health. On the contrary, social ties emerged as critically important, even though individual sociability is not the key. For example, the Terman women outlived the Terman men for a variety of reasons, but especially social reasons, including differing social ties following divorce. As we will see, the real social reasons for long-term health were eye-opening and not what we expected.

· CHAPTER 4 ·

Happiness and Health?
A Cheery Conundrum

In 1922, the parents of the newly enrolled Terman participants were asked to rate their children on how cheerful and optimistic they were, and on their sense of humor. Some were jokesters like Paul, who loved to walk on stilts, roll hoops, and play pom-pom pull away (a game of tag). Others, like Emma, were more mature and serious. Emma loved skating, dancing, and dominoes, but no one would describe her as especially cheerful. The question in our minds, of course, was: Who lived longer, the serious or the cheery?

Many people in our culture peddle the idea that happiness, optimism, and good cheer are the secrets to good health. If true, then if you became ill, you could adopt a positive attitude and recover. It may even help us justify a little too much fun: "Why, dear, I know I am partying heartily tonight, but I need to reduce my stress and maintain my health!" Some scientists have likewise suggested that you can laugh your way to good health. Well, we discovered that happiness and laughter are important, but not for the reasons you might think.

When we looked across the decades at the lives of Paul, Emma, and the other Terman children to see who lived the longest, we found one of the biggest bombshells of our entire project: cheerful and optimistic children were *less* likely to live to an old age than their more staid and sober counterparts!

The finding was no fluke. The magnitude of the detrimental link between cheerfulness and early death was comparable to other known risk factors for mortality such as high blood pressure and high cholesterol. This surprising discovery—that the serious Emmas of the world outlived the cheery Pauls—launched us toward many years of investigation into the relationship between good humor and health. We found that healthy people are happy but happy people are not necessarily healthy. How could this be?

The Cheerful Ones

Terman's cheerful children were those whose parents and teachers reported them to be optimistic and cheerful: "Extraordinarily cheerful and optimistic. Never sees dark side. Never worries." Participants were categorized as having a good sense of humor if the grown-ups in their lives judged them, for example, thus: "Witty. Appreciates jokes. Sees the funny side of everything." Paul, for one, was a fun guy to be around. He laughed often and was rarely ill, only occasionally having a cold. Although he wasn't especially nervous or fearful, his parents felt he was particularly sensitive to the approval and disapproval of others. His parents reported that he slept soundly, usually eight hours per night. They also described him as energetic and sociable, but as more selfish than average. They noted that he "tends to be a leader." Paul and many of the other very cheerful Terman children were not strikingly different from their childhood peers, except for their exceptionally optimistic and fun-loving personalities.

Many people would think that these wags and wits should be less prone to disease, but, as we discovered, such a personality also has its downsides. The experience of joy and other positive emotions can inspire us to do wonderful things in life—raise a child, cooperate with one's team, help someone in need. Good research shows that joyful, engaged individuals are better able to thrive and build positive bonds with others, especially compared to people who are dejected or depressed. But that doesn't mean that going to lively gatherings or swallowing antidepressants will thereby improve health. The real question is: Which comes first, the vigor or the cheer?

Many people believe happiness leads to health because, observably, the two often appear hand in hand—happiness is often associated with health. The correlation has been confirmed as significant in lots of studies, but it does not mean that the happiness is the direct cause of good health. In fact, we have found that in most cases, it is something else—some other set of characteristics—that makes someone both happier and healthier. This distinction is tremendously important because it affects what you should do to maintain and improve health.

Where does some scientific research go wrong? It is easy enough to measure happiness: just ask people (or their friends) how happy or content they feel. In good studies, this assessment is repeated at several times of the day and week.

But how do we assess health? Few researchers are able to follow individuals—those who are very happy, those who are just average, and those who are very sober—for long periods of time to see how long they live and what serious diseases they develop. Instead, they ask subjects, "How healthy are you?" The catch is that people who say they are really happy also are those who are most likely to *say* they are healthy, which tells us nothing about whether their physicians have diagnosed, say, a significant narrowing of their coronary arteries.

Now, the dream scenario would be rigorous studies that made ill individuals happier (through happiness interventions like "counting one's blessings") and then looked to see if they recovered. For example, some individuals with cancer could be scientifically assigned to receive extra treatment and instruction from experts on happiness while a comparison group would receive only the usual cancer treatment. Framed this way, there is very little solid evidence that happiness or good cheer is the panacea that it is often held out to be.[15]

Merriment and Unhealthy Behavior

Is a merry, joyful disposition the mark of great health? Think of our favorite comedians: often they are jocular jesters because they grew up facing very difficult or oppressive situations; they may use humor and joking around to try to cover up trauma or abuse. The upside is that these people have found a way to help themselves cope with severe challenges. The downside is that they have had to experience such obstacles in the first place. Many comedians are, under the surface, grappling with a difficult past. They also tend not to lead the healthiest of lifestyles. Studies of comedians have found that they do not live longer than the rest of us. J. D. Salinger may have been on to something when he wrote, "I'm a kind of paranoiac in reverse. I suspect people of plotting to make me happy."[16]

As we dug in to see why the serious Emmas of the world outlived the cheery Pauls, we considered a number of possibilities.[17] First we looked at what they eventually died from—the causes of death on the certificates that we had collected. Not only were the cheerful Terman participants more likely to die young, we found a hint that the cheerful children were relatively less likely than the average person to die from cancer or heart disease and were instead slightly more likely to die from suicide, accident, or homicide. They also grew up to be more carefree, the "sort who never worry over possible misfortunes," as Dr. Terman put it in 1940. In other words, some of the very cheerful children were either hiding some troubling aspect of their lives or were oblivious to dangers around them. However, we did not find that the cheerful children grew up to be especially poorly adjusted as adults.

We thought that extra health risks might partially be due to something about their daily healthy and unhealthy behaviors. Did the cheerful young children grow up to have poorer habits, perhaps because they were less concerned about things that could go wrong with their bodies? We did find that the Terman children higher on cheerfulness grew up to drink more alcohol and smoke more cigarettes, and vice versa. Emma fit this pattern, as one of the more sober Terman participants who never smoked and reported seldom drinking alcohol. (Maybe it's no coincidence that the word *cheers* is a common toast when clinking alcohol-filled glasses—for individuals on the way to being full of good spirits.)

Did the happy souls actually live life on the edge, seeking out dangerous situations? To find out, we coded their hobbies according to how risky they were. Some participants loved thrilling activities such as aviation and hunting while others preferred safe pastimes such as reading or listening to music. The cheerful children were the ones who grew up to engage in riskier hobbies. Overall, many had a happy-go-lucky disregard for their health. "Put a smile on your face, and lighten up"—cheer up and live long—is another dead-end health myth.

At this point, we knew that something complicated was going on: there are positive aspects of being cheerful and happy, but there are negative, threatening aspects as well. We burrowed deeper into the matter, probing both the later lives of the Terman participants and the relevant research of other investigators.

The Tinker Bell Principle

The idea that optimism and good cheer are the secret to health is especially appealing to those who are ill. The more serious and challenging the disease, the more we hope for a mind-to-body effect in which good thoughts yield vigor and vitality. We have named this the Tinker Bell Principle, after the character in *Peter Pan* whose survival depends on enough people believing in fairies.

There is certainly good evidence for what is sometimes called mind over matter, when it involves focusing your attention on other things to cope with pain or minor troubles. But could optimism actually shrink a tumor or open a clogged artery? And if so, how can we increase our optimism?

One strategy for promoting or reinforcing optimism in sick persons is to give them placebos. Sugar pills, "magnetic" therapy, and even going to exorcists do "work" sometimes.[18] In fact, they often work well (even in controlled scientific studies) for about one-third of people, especially when the problem is pain or a test of endurance in the face of a difficult treatment. As we noted, the more challenging question is whether optimism and placebos can help cure those with serious diseases.

Being optimistic or believing in a placebo treatment does affect the body's physiology to some extent, but there is little firm evidence that this in itself will rev up the immune system enough to provide miracle cures. Instead, one clue to placebo effectiveness lies in the fact that optimistic people expect that their futures will be full of positive outcomes—that their labors will work out for the best. This means that optimistic people are more willing to persist in their efforts and stick with their goals, even when they encounter obstacles or adversity. If their families are likewise optimistic, so much the better. It's easy to imagine how this attitude would help someone facing a complex prescribed medical regimen, a painful rehabilitation, or chemotherapy.

In other words, the main impact of optimism on health is that it encourages health-promoting behaviors. For someone who is seriously ill, this might mean an extra push to drink some water and get out of bed. For someone facing a chronic condition like HIV, it might mean taking all those pills on time, cutting out alcohol, or seeing the best doctors one can possibly find. Optimists like Paul are generally better at coping with challenges in the short term, a trait that can help one through a medical emergency. For example, Paul's successful battle with pneumonia when he was forty-two was seemingly aided by the optimistic belief that he would surely recover—which encouraged him to stick with the regimen his doctor recommended, including uncomfortable and tedious breathing exercises.

Furthermore, if patients feel reassured after getting a placebo treatment, they're more likely to sleep and eat better. Their stress levels will be lower and their bodies will have a better shot at reestablishing inner balance. Even if poor nutrition or stress weren't the root cause of the illness, an optimistic motivation could provide the needed impetus for corrective actions.

However, the long-term effects of high levels of optimism (and cheerfulness) are not necessarily beneficial. If you are facing serious surgery and a long recovery, then realistic optimism is good. It may enable you to get on your feet faster and go home from the hospital sooner. But too much optimism can leave you surprised, disappointed, and seriously frustrated with any unexpected long-term hardships. Moderate worriers would actually do better in such situations—more on that later.

Tinker Bell recovers, but unfortunately we see no good evidence for the pure and simple form of this approach—that if you and your supportive friends think good thoughts, you'll thereby get better. There is some evidence for a more sophisticated version of this idea, though, in which people who are optimistic at the right times and to the right degree will remain healthier and live longer.

In a bit we'll explain how we uncovered a helpful role for worrying.

Illusory Optimism and Those Most Senior of Citizens

A significant health downside to optimism involves overlooking or ignoring real threats—sometimes called illusory optimism. Optimistic people, like happy people, may underestimate risks to their health and thereby fail to take precautions or to follow medical advice. The same optimistic thoughts that may promote recovery from surgery ("I'm going to be just fine") may prove deadly to a cigarette smoker, a hypertensive, or an overeater.

Or, optimistic people may be especially shocked when things turn out badly. So they experience additional stress in the face of a job loss, a death in the family, or the return of cancer. Not only that, but they may then resume life-threatening habits.[19]

But don't the oldest of the old, in the most golden of the golden years, tend to have a positive outlook? Studies of centenarians do find that long-lived people are optimistic. But this line of research has a serious flaw: there's no proper comparison group. People who live to be one hundred have an affirmative view on life, but compared to whom? Maybe it was the grouches at age fifty who, after thriving for another half century, became the centenarians with the positive outlook. In fact, who wouldn't feel rosy in front of a birthday cake aglow with one hundred candles?

This flaw in the centenarian research helps explain why so many of the findings of past studies on the secrets to longevity rarely hold up. Eat all the yogurt you can stand, and you are still very unlikely to reach a hundred. In our analyses of the Terman participants, we do look at those who reached extreme old age, but we do so in the context of their full lives, from childhood on. And in fact, studies (by other scientists) on mood and aging find that as adults get older, they generally are happier and experience fewer negative emotions.[20] The oldest among us are happy, but the happiness did not cause their long lives.

Would other research projects confirm this line of thinking? Aside from Dr. Terman's project, there are only a few other excellent studies capable of looking at these matters of happiness and health in the proper way. One of the best is the Harvard Study of Adult Development, which has followed about 250 men since they were in college at Harvard in the 1930s. This study has found that men who coped with life's challenges in a mature manner and maintained deep social relationships fared best. These men tended to have stable marriages and healthy habits (avoiding smoking and alcohol abuse and staying trim). Especially relevant to our own work on happiness and health is one of the most insightful conclusions by the head investigator of the Harvard study, Dr. George Vaillant, who contrasts the "Happy-Well" with the "Sad-Sick."[21] Some paths led the Harvard men to be happy and well while other paths led to being sad and sick. Happiness was not the cause of wellness. Sadness was not the cause of sickness. Instead, Vaillant concluded, happiness or sadness was an *outcome*, just as was wellness or sickness.

Dr. David Snowdon has been running another rare long-term study—the Nun Study—that has information on about seven hundred women across many decades. Needless to say, the nuns, of the School Sisters of Notre Dame, were not smokers, drinkers, or sexual adventurers. They had adequate housing, medical care, and social relations. Yet they did show individual differences.[22] Those with higher verbal skills, more education, and positive emotions in young adulthood did better and lived longer. The young women who expressed more hope and gratitude in their diaries went on to live healthier lives than those revealing sadness and fear. But some nuns showed dips and declines in their moods, language, *and* health. Happiness and health often shifted in parallel. For example, those who would eventually develop Alzheimer's disease articulated less and less positive emotion as their mental functions got worse and worse. Surely their poor moods were not causing their rapid mental decline.

We thus needed to understand much more about grumpiness, happiness, and anxiety across long periods of time. So we next turned our attention directly to issues of mood, worrying, and mental health across the decades.

Are Neurotic Individuals Unhealthy?

Fidgety Philip was moody, tense, and high-strung. Full of "tireless" energy, he was well liked by his schoolmates despite tending to seek the attention of others through his behaviors. Philip was not especially conscientious, applying himself diligently only to tasks that interested him. His mother noted that he was more nervous than the average child, prone to worry about many things including burglars and being alone. In 1922, the Terman subjects' parents and teachers rated them on how moody they were. Were their moods very changeable—that is, often alternating between joy and sadness? Or were they more decidedly stable and permanent? Philip's mother responded, "moods extremely changeable," when describing her son. Dr. Terman thought that these reactions might be relevant to their later lives, and he turned out to be correct.

As we consistently found with our Terman studies, answers never wrapped up neatly. So while moodiness often had a negative impact on health and longevity, sometimes this worrying nature helped out later in life. In 1940, the Terman subjects were about thirty years old. Philip, it turns out, had grown up to be quite a worrier. Now married, he was the proud father of a daughter, but he remained moody and cared a good deal about what others thought of him. James, too, was rather anxious and uptight, but in a more focused way. A sensitive child, he'd become a sensitive adult, frequently keyed-up and restless, worrying about his financial planning and various other hassles of living through turbulent times. Although these characteristics were telling, we wanted to create a more formal measure of what scientists term *neuroticism*—the tendency to worry and be moody, tense, and at risk of rage or depression. We needed a scale that was reliable and valid, and so we sorted through dozens of Terman's questionnaire items, scrutinized how they related to each other, and used advanced statistical analysis to extract items for a reliable scale. We then validated the scale against modern measures of neuroticism.

SELF-ASSESSMENT: NEUROTICISM

Here is a self-assessment scale that yields some insight into the relationship between moody worrying and longevity.

Are you very affected by praise or blame?	3 – Yes 2 – ? 1 – No
Do you often feel just miserable?	3 – Yes 2 – ? 1 – No
Are you touchy on certain topics?	3 – Yes 2 – ? 1 – No
Does some particularly useless thought keep coming into your mind to bother you?	3 – Yes 2 – ? 1 – No

Are you frequently burdened by a sense of remorse or regret?	3 – Yes 2 – ? 1 – No
Do you worry too long over humiliating experiences?	3 – Yes 2 – ? 1 – No
Do your feelings alternate between happiness and sadness without apparent reason?	3 – Yes 2 – ? 1 – No
Are your feelings easily hurt?	3 – Yes 2 – ? 1 – No
Are you moody?	3 – Yes 2 – ? 1 – No
Do you tend to be quite emotional?	3 – Yes 2 – ? 1 – No

To score this quiz, do the following. For each of the ten questions, assign a score of 3 for "yes," 1 for "no," and 2 for any question mark that you circled. Now add up your total score. The lowest possible score is 10 and highest possible is 30. If you scored 18 or below you are clearly a relaxed, laid-back kind of person—you are in the bottom quartile of this neuroticism scale, based on our data. If your score is 23 or above, however, you're something of a neurotic (you are scoring in the upper quartile).

The term "neurotic" here isn't being used in the clinical sense but rather to describe a normal personality characteristic that everyone possesses to one degree or another. If you scored in the middle, you are probably rather high-strung at times and appear a bit neurotic, but at other times you are more calm and serene.

When It's Okay to Worry

As young and middle-aged adults, the Terman participants were asked whether they were generally in a good mood, calm and relaxed, and satisfied with their lives. We also knew whether, late in life, they reported declining health, a heart condition, cancer, or difficulty in completing daily tasks without assistance. Emma (who was serious as a child), for example, was retired and living alone, but said she was happy—at the time of her report she estimated that she had been "fairly cheerful" and "fairly relaxed" over the prior couple of months. She had successfully battled breast cancer not long after her retirement, remained energetic, and even did a bit of traveling from time to time. Her health story was typical of some but contrasted with other Terman subjects, who needed considerable help to care for themselves, were anxious and depressed, or saw their lives as "not too happy."

When we homed in on adult personality, later-life happiness, and health and longevity, we found that the Terman women who were worriers in young adulthood went on to later report being sicker and unhappier; and they were more likely to die at a younger age. This was especially true if they were not prudent and conscientious. If the women were conscientious and in control of their lives and had a good group of friends, then their worrying proved to be much less of a health threat.

For men, the results were dramatically different. The Terman men who were worriers in young adulthood went on to later report being sicker and unhappier on average, but they were *less* likely to die. If the neurotic individuals were also conscientious, things got even better. The men who were conscientious *and* neurotic, like James, did quite well as they aged—at least in terms of their length of life. Older men who are neurotic worriers may be especially motivated to take care of themselves, in part due to a preoccupation with bodily symptoms.

Rather than fretting themselves to death, they are concerned enough to keep themselves alive.

At first we were a bit suspicious of this clear but unexpected benefit to neurotic men, though it is hard to argue with death certificates. But then two studies by other researchers appeared, finding the same pattern. One showed that elderly men (over age seventy) who were neurotic were less likely to die during the next four years, and the other, a study of elderly Medicare patients, found that neuroticism was health protective.[23] We also became believers when we saw that our discovery was especially true of the Terman men who were widowed—a time when it becomes especially important to take care of oneself.

We will come back to the dramatic differences we found between men and women, especially bereaved men and women, later on in the book. The lesson for now is that there are definitely times when it is very healthy to be a worrier.

Are You Agreeable?

If you are friendly, cooperative, trusting, and kind, then psychologists would label your personality as *agreeable*. This dimension—agreeableness—does a good job of summarizing the differences people have in how supportive and helpful they are. To measure the Terman participants in this way, we turned to questions they had answered about themselves in young adulthood—things like whether they tried to avoid arguments, were not critical of others, avoided hurting others' feelings, paid attention to the feelings of others, and didn't always try to get their own way. When describing herself in 1940, Emma indicated that she was not likely to "upbraid a workman who fail[ed] to have work done on time" nor was she likely to lose her temper, criticize others, or ignore their feelings. Instead, she saw herself as someone who was "easy to get on with." She scored quite high on our measure of agreeableness.

While our study confirmed what other good research has shown—that agreeable, altruistic people are happier and tend to remain that way—simply being agreeable was not a secret to long life. There was certainly indication that agreeable folks stayed healthier, especially in terms of having good social relationships. But it was the social relationships themselves that turned out to be more important to physical health and long life. Being agreeable predisposed Emma to make friends and do for others but was not a direct link to her health. We'd discovered yet another case of how the importance of happiness to health is often overstated or misinterpreted. People involved in social and altruistic activities tend to be happy. But making a person happy and cheery will not necessarily make them altruistic and involved in charitable activities.

Just as worrying is not necessarily bad for your health, being agreeable is not always good for your health; it all depends on where you are on your life's pathway and what situations you're currently facing. That's not to say that emotions aren't relevant to health; rather it means you have to be a little more sophisticated and do a little more thinking about how these emotions matter for your individual case.

Shared Paths to Health and Happiness

Really tall people purchase clothes that are sized as "extra long," but few of us would buy extra long clothes in an effort to make ourselves grow taller. Sometimes it is very clear that there are underlying causes, such as genes and good nutrition, that lead to the association between two results. Yet in the health field, we constantly go astray in our understanding of what causes what.

One of our colleagues and friends is the distinguished researcher Sonja Lyubomirsky. Sonja is a leader in studying interventions that make people happier. One day, looking over the recommendations that Sonja and other happiness researchers make about improving and maintaining happiness, we were struck by an amazing correspondence and connection: many (but not all) of the recommendations for happiness are nearly identical to recommendations for maintaining health.

For example, those trying to improve their happiness are advised to do the following things:

- Watch less TV
- Improve social relations—spend time with friends
- Increase levels of physical activity—go for a long walk
- Help others and express gratitude to those who have helped you
- Take on new challenges to remain fresh and in-the-moment

These are all connected to health and long life, but we view them differently and would reframe the process: rather than recommending that you do each of these items, our research with the Terman participants suggests finding a lifestyle in which doing each of these things comes naturally. That is, these recommended activities are part of long-term patterns that characterize healthy and happy individuals. The healthy patterns and pathways come first, and they lead to both health and happiness.

What It Means for You: Guideposts to Health and Long Life

Let's face it, if you hear advice to stop watching your favorite television shows, put away your snacks, and go out running, you are very unlikely to do it. If you are really motivated, you might try for a while but then soon enough fall back into your old habits. But if you are the kind of person who is really, really busy with friends, family, congregation, a sports league, a challenging career, travel, book clubs, and more, then you won't have much time to sit, snack, and watch TV.

The same is true of an artificial attempt to express gratitude to your mentors. It works (at cheering you up) in the short term but then falls by the wayside, unless it strengthens social bonds. The Terman subjects who were very happy (and many were very happy) never received formal instruction about happiness. They did not live in a land of laugh therapy, self-esteem clinics, and indulgent parents.[24] Instead, they traveled pathways of living that made them happy, healthy, (often) wealthy, and wise.

In fact, many knew that being happy is not the same as being healthy, and that worrying is sometimes a *good* thing. The Terman participants who lived long happy lives were not cynical rebels and loners. They were indeed accomplished individuals who were satisfied with their lives, but they did not pursue happiness. They were happy and laughed *because* they were healthy, wealthy, and wise—their happiness was a by-product of their pathways to long life. As we shall see, their particular types of social relations, careers, hobbies, and habits paved the true royal road to health.

So the reason that healthy people like Emma are happy but happy people are not necessarily healthy is that living a certain lifestyle puts you on the paths to long life that simultaneously make you happy and fulfilled; but cheering yourself up with short-term pleasures will usually do nothing remarkable for your health. Emma was not an especially cheery and optimistic child, but that didn't interfere with her later health and happiness. If you find friends who laugh with you, then that is probably a healthy thing. If you find television shows that make you laugh all evening while you sit alone and eat, then that is not healthy. "Cheer up and live long" is much too simple—another dead-end myth.

If the same things that lead to happiness often lead to health, and the same things that improve health also boost happiness, then it should not be terribly surprising that happier folks are healthier or that tall folks wear extra long clothes. Sometimes, improving your health may improve your happiness. Sometimes, in facing very troubling times, happy people can cope well and maintain their health. But mostly, doing the right things will improve both your happiness and your health.

· CHAPTER 5 ·

Catastrophic Thinking

The Fates of Chicken Littles

If an acorn drops on your head and you conclude that the sky is falling, psychologists might call you a "catastrophizer." There is a pattern to how people explain or interpret bad events: catastrophizers see impending doom everywhere, while sunnier types are quick to see signs of fortune in their midst. If you are the former, you might really have something to fear: this pattern may be a forewarning of increased mortality risk.

We decided to explore how the Terman subjects viewed and explained the world when they were young adults, and specifically how their degree of catastrophizing might influence the length of their lives and the cause of their deaths.

Chicken Little Meets Content Analysis

Catastrophizing is expressed not so much in how people feel about events or how they respond, but in how they *think* about things that happen or may happen to them. The bad part is that catastrophizers—the Chicken Littles of the world who think the sky is falling—can bring trouble onto themselves. The good news is that catastrophizing involves your thoughts, and thoughts can be changed and improved.

For this part of the longevity project, we collaborated with Professors Chris Peterson and Martin Seligman, experts in *explanatory style*—how individuals explain the causes of bad happenings. For example, some people tend to blame themselves when something goes wrong, rather than putting the onus on someone else or on bad luck. Some individuals also see difficulties as more permanent or long lasting than is justified. They think, "This problem is going to last forever!"

Most important, some individuals overgeneralize the problem: instead of seeing it as limited and specific, they believe it is going to undermine everything they do. Their life is "a total mess." These are the true catastrophizers—their pessimistic view of life sees every stumble as a calamity. Karen was like this. She was timid and had little self-confidence, even in childhood, and was described in grade school as extraordinarily sensitive to the disapproval of others. Her teacher noted that, when disciplined, she took it hard and seemed to have difficulty getting over the experience. At about that same time her mother reported that Karen had persistent fears of being kidnapped. In short, Karen's perception of her life seemed to be that one bad thing would follow another.

When they were in their late twenties, the subjects wrote answers to Dr. Terman's questions about their own flaws and about the bad events they had faced. In particular, they were asked about their most serious faults of personality or character to date. They were also asked to describe disappointments, failures, bereavements, and unfriendly relationships with others that had a prolonged influence on them. Some noted minor flaws of character, such as being too ambitious or too painstaking. Others, such as Karen, had gone through the divorce of their parents and lost all faith in the possibility of happy marriage. Some were harsh in their self-criticism: Karen vividly described her shyness and its effect on her life, something she saw as an insurmountable character flaw.

Our research collaborators, using a technique called content analysis, analyzed and coded the explanations that the Terman participants had written. That is, trained reviewers evaluated to what extent each person was a catastrophizer in early adulthood, based on criteria such as the vocabulary they used. They reviewed over 3,000 such explanations from almost 1,200 participants, then shipped the evaluations to us, and we conducted the complicated statistical analyses needed to determine if there was a connection between a catastrophic outlook and longevity.

Catastrophizing and Mortality

The results were clear. The catastrophizers died sooner. The difference was especially large for the men.[25] This held true even if we excluded anyone who died in the five years immediately following the assessment, ruling out the possibility that a participant was already seriously ill and influenced by his or her predicament.

Catastrophizers generally have superficial relationships with other people and cannot face their problems.[26] Fidgety Philip was one of the worst Terman study catastrophizers. He viewed his misfortunes as pervasive in their effects—seeing his character flaws as qualities that permeated every aspect of his life. (He described his impulsiveness and inability to control his alcohol use as being his two biggest faults.) Like Karen, Philip interpreted each of his misfortunes as bigger than life. He died of a heart attack before his sixty-fifth birthday.

Catastrophizing-Related Ailments: How They Died

Why did so many of the catastrophizers die young? We found a relevant source of information in the death certificates. We grouped the causes of death into four categories: cardiovascular disease (heart attacks or strokes), cancer, accidents or violence (homicide, suicide, car crashes, and so on), and "other" causes, such as infection.

Catastrophizers were clearly more likely to die from accidents or violence. But they were only slightly more likely (than noncatastrophizers) to die from the various other causes of death. So we had a good clue as to why catastrophizing was especially deadly—it's dangerous. People who believe that having one significant problem is a sign that lots and lots of bad things will follow put themselves onto risky paths, especially in terms of the likelihood of a violent early death. They blamed themselves for far too much and they suffered the consequences. This was poignantly true in Karen's case. She took her own life while still in her thirties.

Yet not all catastrophizers, nor even most catastrophizers, faced the fate of an early demise. Many improved their viewpoint over time and then changed the direction of their lives. Nevertheless, how people explained the world around them turned out to be one predictive piece in the longevity puzzle.

SELF-ASSESSMENT: CATASTROPHIZING

Below, circle the response that best reflects how true each statement is of you.

1. I worry that life will get worse and worse.

  5 – very accurate
  4 – moderately accurate
  3 – neither accurate nor inaccurate
  2 – moderately inaccurate
  1 – very inaccurate

2. When I look at the state of the world, I see opportunities everywhere.

  5 – very accurate
  4 – moderately accurate
  3 – neither accurate nor inaccurate
  2 – moderately inaccurate
  1 – very inaccurate

3. I have a magic touch—when I get involved in an issue everything seems to work out fine.

  5 – very accurate
  4 – moderately accurate
  3 – neither accurate nor inaccurate
  2 – moderately inaccurate
  1 – very inaccurate

4. I routinely blow my chances and mess up my opportunities.

5 – very accurate
4 – moderately accurate
3 – neither accurate nor inaccurate
2 – moderately inaccurate
1 – very inaccurate

5. I fear that the worst is going to happen.

5 – very accurate
4 – moderately accurate
3 – neither accurate nor inaccurate
2 – moderately inaccurate
1 – very inaccurate

6. When I mess up on little things, other things start falling apart.

5 – very accurate
4 – moderately accurate
3 – neither accurate nor inaccurate
2 – moderately inaccurate
1 – very inaccurate

Scoring: For statements 2 and 3, which are phrased in the opposite direction, reverse your scores (that is, if you gave yourself a 5 change it to a 1, change a 4 to a 2, leave 3 as it is, change a 2 to a 4, and replace a 1 with a 5. Now add up your score—it should fall between 6 and 30. An average score on this catastrophizing scale is about 12 or 13; those who are particularly mellow about mishaps will score below 10, whereas definite catastrophizers will score at 24 or higher.

The Mysterious End of Douglas Kelley

Douglas McGlashan Kelley—one of the publicly identified Terman participants—was also one of the most interesting and baffling. Kelley grew up in San Francisco, was discovered by Dr. Terman for his study, and went to college at the University of California in Berkeley. He became a well-known psychiatrist and a Berkeley professor. He was an energetic and well-adjusted child, though less conscientious than most. Although Kelley was empathic and sensitive to the feelings of others, there was nothing remarkable in his childhood that would portend the dramatic turns his life would take.

Douglas Kelley loved jokes and magic. In fact, in 1941 *Time* magazine featured him in an article as a psychiatrist who taught parlor tricks to his patients. In 1942, at age twenty-nine, Dr. Kelley was called to the U.S. Army Medical Corps and sent to Europe to serve as a forensic psychiatrist, his specialty. When the war ended, he received a unique assignment. He was attached to the International Military Tribunal in Nuremberg, Germany, where Nazi war crimes trials were being prepared. His job was to study some of the highest-ranking captured Nazis, including the foreign minister Joachim von Ribbentrop, and Hermann Goering, one of the most infamous and powerful Nazis.

Dr. Kelley administered psychological assessments such as the Rorschach inkblot test to the imprisoned Nazi leaders. Kelley was a Rorschach expert. Fascinated with their views, he also spent many hours talking with them, trying to understand how they could commit such awful crimes against fellow human beings. He decided that the Nazi leaders were mentally competent to stand trial. Eventually Von Ribbentrop and other top Nazis were hanged, but Hermann Goering secretly swallowed potassium cyanide the night before he was to be executed.

After the war Douglas Kelley became a criminologist as well as a professor. He testified in court about the mental state of those accused of crimes, similar to his work in Nuremberg. He even broke new ground in the psychiatric use of drugs like Sodium Pentothal as a potential truth serum. Dr. Kelley wrote a book called *22 Cells in Nuremberg*. Oddly, he also collected Nazi memorabilia.

On New Year's Day in 1958, Douglas Kelley suddenly killed himself at home in front of his family. He was just forty-five years old. His method of suicide was striking: Dr. Kelley killed himself by swallowing cyanide. The next day, the *New York Times* quoted police as saying that the poison capsule "was one of several souvenir capsules Dr. Kelley had brought home from Nuremberg. The capsules had been discovered on Hermann W. Goering, who committed suicide by taking a similar capsule on October 16, 1946, two hours before he was scheduled to be hanged."[27]

No one ever figured out for sure why Douglas Kelley, a successful doctor, suddenly killed himself, leaving a loving wife and three young children. (Paradoxically, in a memorial tribute to Kelley after his death, his colleagues at the University of California wrote of "his characteristically jovial humor.") But a reasonable guess would be that as a young adult, he came to know that something about the world was terribly wrong. A sensitive person forced to face the worst of human horrors up close, he would come to see many things as far more ominous and catastrophic than would the average person. He knew firsthand how evil and scheming even educated individuals could be. Although he was outwardly successful for years after this life-changing experience, his sense of order, agency, and meaning had been shattered.

The Terman Women Who Ended It All

Our collaborator Carol Tomlinson-Keasey spearheaded a fascinating investigation of suicide, focused on eight women in the Terman sample who were definitively confirmed to have killed themselves.[28] There may well have been additional suicides among the Terman women—some of the additional deaths by drug overdose were probably really suicides and not accidents. But the strongest conclusions can be made by examining those who had "suicide" listed as the cause of death on their certificates, or who had left suicide notes.

Men generally prefer guns or other violent means for taking their own lives, whereas women often turn to drugs. More than half of the confirmed female suicides among the Terman participants were by drug overdose (most often by a fatal dose of barbiturates), but there was also the occasional gunshot and carbon monoxide poisoning. Most of the suicides occurred when the women were in the prime of life—between thirty and forty-four years old. What would have led these very bright women to kill themselves? Was it an attempt to escape constant pain, anxiety, or depression by departing to a better place? Was it a very moody, impulsive temperament that led to a spur-of-the-moment decision to end it all? Was it sparked by the loss of a loved one in their lives?

In order to determine which factors were most relevant to suicide, proper comparison groups were needed. One was a matched group of women from the Terman sample who had died at the same ages (within one year) as the suicides, but from natural causes. This matched group allowed an evaluation of the typical life path of someone who died of cancer, for example, as compared to someone who swallowed a bottle of sleeping pills.

The second comparison group consisted of randomly selected female Terman subjects who lived at least until 1964, the year when the last of the scrutinized suicides occurred. This group allowed investigation into whether there might be some factors that distinguished women who died prematurely—whether by suicide or by illness—from women who survived into later life.

When we do exploratory research of this type, we want to find the relevant predictors, but we don't want to capitalize on chance and find what was just a random quirk, never to be found again. The problem is, the more comparisons you make, the more likely you are to find some differences that came about only by chance and aren't meaningful. That is, if researchers compare thousands of variables across the three groups of Terman participants—suicides, early natural deaths, and those who lived into later life—they would find some variables that differ substantially between the groups just by chance. To avoid this, the solution is to focus on aspects and characteristics, dealt with in other studies, that are either suspected or known to be associated with suicide.

The first of those variables is physical health. The next is stress: for this the researchers used a measure of childhood stress, a measure of adulthood stress, a coding of whether the participant had lost her father before she was twenty (a known risk factor for girls' mental health), and a mental health index developed by Dr. Terman and his coinvestigator Melita Oden. Then came a combined measure of temperament: in 1940, were the women reporting that they were moody, unhappy, impulsive, emotional, lacking self-confidence, or feeling inferior? Finally, the researchers applied scores for what the suicidologist Edwin Shneidman called signatures of suicide—relevant elements of mental health that increase the risk of suicide. These include depression, substance abuse, anxiety, instability, and past attempted suicide.

These potential suicide predictors were then used in a statistical procedure called discriminant function analysis. The Internal Revenue Service uses discriminant function analysis to predict whether you may be a tax cheat, based on various elements of your tax return as well as previous knowledge of past cheaters. In the case of Terman suicides, this type of analysis is used to measure which elements of one's history and pathway may predict willingness to cheat life.

The signatures of suicidal mental health did an impressive job of predicting whether someone would commit suicide, have an early natural death, or live a long life. In addition, high levels of stress and a moody, impulsive temperament contributed to the risk.

Most interesting, however, was that individual characteristics, things about the social environment, *and* challenges relevant to stress *all* contributed to suicide risk. It wasn't just anxiety and depression, it wasn't just alcoholism, it wasn't just early life stress, and it wasn't just instability in relationships and careers. All of these things mattered—a person's overall pathway influenced the likelihood of suicide.

Many Terman subjects, for example, were anxious or faced serious challenges but lived long lives. It was those who ignored the guideposts to good health who were most at risk—they traveled down pathways that became more and more dangerous, and eventually fatal. On the other hand, those who circled back to the healthy road often went on to a long life.

Terman Men Who Shot Themselves

The late suicidologist Dr. Shneidman did not think too highly of blaming suicide on a chemical imbalance in the brain. He knew that suicide was related to deeper issues surrounding the meaning of life and death, and he knew that suicide rates varied greatly across cultures, times, and circumstances. He concluded that it couldn't be fully understood as a brain disease, nor fully prevented with antidepressant drugs. He did not use the term *catastrophizing*, but he knew and agreed that the ways people thought about the world were keys to understanding suicide.

One day Dr. Shneidman called us; he started to identify himself, but we knew who he was. We knew that in addition to his other groundbreaking work, Shneidman had studied the lives of five Terman men who had shot themselves while still in their forties or fifties.[29]

As with the study of Terman women, this project also used two control groups—men who died at comparable ages from illness, and men who lived long lives. In a clever research move, Dr. Shneidman had an assistant prepare detailed biographies of each of the men, from childhood through about age thirty, but with all information about the man's subsequent longevity removed. (For example, in one prepared biography, a high school counselor had written that the young man was emotionally unstable and morally erratic, while a Terman staffer who had visited the same subject described more details and reported that he was quite likable.) Shneidman then carefully read the materials in each man's folder, without knowing which group the man was in, that is, without seeing his eventual fate. Unbeknownst to Shneidman, five were suicides by gunshot, ten were natural deaths at a comparable age, and fifteen were men still living.

Dr. Shneidman evaluated each of these Terman participants on two dimensions. The first was one he called "perturbation," a measure of the person's level of agitation, disturbance, and lack of composure. This measure included a focus on the man's early relationships with his parents; his level of life success or failure; and the presence of the markers of poor mental health, such as alcoholism, depression, and instability.

Shneidman's second dimension was something he called "lethality," which included features of the man's life that reflected his likely intentions about his death. This could be recent anticipations of trouble, thoughts or premonitions of accidents or death, or disappointments with accomplishments. (One of the Terman subjects, for example, reported at age twenty-nine that he now believed that his early intellectual gifts had been merely a flash in the pan.) After reviewing the prepared biographies, and evaluating perturbation and lethality, Shneidman used his clinical judgment to rank the thirty men included in his analysis in order of the likelihood of their suicide.

Dr. Shneidman's accuracy was striking. His rankings placed all five of the actual suicides in his top six most likely suicides. He was not using numeric data put through a discriminant analysis, as was done in the study of female Terman suicides, but his clinical judgments were correct. He was able to capture those aspects of the men's lives that foretold their later suicide.

The men who shot themselves thought that something important was missing in their lives. They drew from that a bigger conclusion—that their lives were not worth living. In addition to their unstable lives, their disappointment in their achievements—the discrepancy between what they aspired to do and what they actually accomplished—weighed very heavily on these men, and they believed all was lost. These beliefs are very similar to the catastrophizing that our studies have shown to correlate more broadly with early death from violent causes.

By the way, it is interesting to note that when Dr. Shneidman was not studying suicide, he was studying the novels and essays of the dark romance novelist Herman Melville. He especially loved *Moby-Dick*. Whenever the protagonist in *Moby-Dick* feels a damp, drizzly November in his soul and involuntarily pauses before coffin warehouses, it is high time to get to sea as soon as he can. But in real life, Melville's own son Malcolm shot himself and died. Shneidman, Melville, and Douglas Kelley shared a fascination with the deeper existential issues of catastrophizing thoughts.

Thoughts in Old Age

The reason Ed Shneidman had telephoned us was that he had learned of our ongoing work with the Terman participants, and he wanted to send us the audiotapes of the in-depth interviews he had conducted with Terman men late in life—in the 1980s—when both he and the subjects were over age seventy. Dr. Shneidman was living in Los Angeles, as were forty-five of the Terman men. He saw the men every year or so through 1987 (about seven years), mostly asking them about their lives. One particularly fascinating report he wrote focused on eleven of these Terman men who were lawyers (or retired lawyers).

Shneidman transcribed all the interview responses of these eleven participants, across fifty-one interview sessions and 241,985 words. He analyzed the frequencies of all the words they used in their responses to his open-ended questions. He felt their vocabulary would provide some insight into how these aging men thought about their lives.

The men who were in this group were generally successful and relatively healthy for their age. Most were still working (at least part-time) into their seventies and early eighties. We knew that catastrophizing tended to predict who would die prematurely, but what thought style was predominant among those who aged successfully?

Perhaps not surprisingly, these older men, who were still able and eager to contribute to society, willing to participate in Shneidman's interviews, and capable of reflecting on their lives, did not sound like catatastrophizers at all. The most prominent conversation topics—based both on the number of different words used and on the total number of occurrences of words related to that topic—were occupation, family, and health.

But then came a bombshell of an insight: over all the interviews with these older men (almost a quarter of a million words), not a single man ever spoke the word *death* in reference to his own inevitable demise. A few times they used the word *death* when mentioning the recent death of a friend, but mostly they talked about their work and their families. Some talked a great deal about their health (and about their own efforts and the efforts of their doctors to maintain their health), but their utterances revealed that they did not focus on death. They talked about their lives, not about their deaths.

Does this mean that the secret to long life is making sure never to talk about death? Not any more than the secret to long life is watching funny TV shows. The ways the long-lived Terman participants thought about and interpreted their lives were part of their healthy patterns, patterns that developed and deepened over many years.

Any Regrets?

In 1986, when the Terman participants who were still alive were about seventy-five years old, they filled out a questionnaire that included an open-ended question: "What choices would you make differently if you had the opportunity to live life again?" Their answers provide further insight into the thinking of the participants, as they looked back over their lives. Researchers at Cornell University performed one detailed analysis of these answers.[30]

Dr. Shneidman's work had revealed that the discrepancy between what the Terman men aspired to do professionally and what they actually did weighed very heavily on the men who were contemplating (and eventually committed) suicide. Would the Terman participants who lived to old age therefore have few regrets? The septuagenarian Terman participants' responses in 1986 were coded in terms of whether the regrets—the things they wished they had done differently—were mostly about actions they had taken. Examples of commonly regretted actions were marrying too young, smoking and drinking too much, and focusing too much on career. Or were they okay with what they had done but concerned about actions they had *failed* to take? Commonly regretted inactions were not completing college or graduate school, not working hard enough in school, not aiming high enough in their career, and not emphasizing social relationships enough.

It turned out that there was a very strong predominance of regretting inactions—opportunities lost—over regretting actions. Rather than thinking about whether they had worked too hard on their careers, they wondered about other careers they might have enjoyed.

In other words, the individuals in this late-life sample of Terman participants were reflecting generally positive thoughts about life.

These older men had survived to their midseventies in good enough physical and mental health to be filling out questionnaires. When they looked back over their lives, they didn't perceive that things had turned out so badly for them—for the most part, as life went on, they didn't regret what they had done. But they thought that their lives could have been even better if they had taken even further advantage of the opportunities they had confronted.

Conscientiousness and Catastrophizing

By this point in our studies of Karen, Douglas Kelley, Philip, and all the other Terman participants, we knew that conscientiousness was a major factor in long life. But did conscientiousness relate to catastrophizing and the associated early deaths? It did. The conscientious participants were less likely to be the catastrophizers. In fact, even when symptoms of mental illness in early adulthood were held constant, the children who had been more conscientiousness were less likely to commit suicide.[31]

One reason conscientious individuals live longer is that they cooperate with their medical treatments. Though not surprising, this is important. People who don't take their pills in the manner that their doctors prescribe them (such as three times a day with food), or who don't even bother to take their pills at all, are obviously less likely to have a successful medical treatment. In fact, very large numbers of patients—millions in the United States alone—do not cooperate well with their doctors. Sometimes they can't afford the treatments, and sometimes they find the treatments too uncomfortable to endure. Sometimes they dislike their doctors.

But many such failures to comply are due to personality. Some people simply do not bother to fully understand their treatments or follow directions. Or they believe that they are doomed in any case: after becoming ill, they catastrophize that everything is over. They are unconscientious, imprudent, and unmotivated.

There is a startling twist, however, to the importance of conscientiousness and noncatastrophizing that is not well understood even by most doctors. The pervasive effects of conscientiousness on health go well beyond these cooperation effects (also called adherence effects).

An excellent randomized study conducted a number of years ago at Yale University on medication use after a heart attack well illustrates this point.[32] Patients were given either the medication Propranolol or a placebo sugar pill. The researchers then followed the patients to see who would live long and who would die. What is remarkable about this study is that researchers also evaluated how well each of the participants cooperated with the treatment and took their pills. This was an especially unusual step at the time.

Their first finding was valuable news to cardiologists but not so interesting to us: patients who did not cooperate well with their prescribed treatment—that is, who took less than 75 percent of the prescribed pills—were more than two times more likely to die within a year of follow-up than patients who took all their pills. After all, how could the pills help you if you do not take them?

Most interesting to us, however, was that the conscientious patients (the good adherers) were much more likely to survive whether they were on the Propranolol medication or on the placebo. Being conscientious enough—adherent enough—to fully cooperate with treatment, even if with a placebo, emerged as a more important predictor of mortality risk than the medication itself. Their overall approach to life was what mattered most, not the drug per se.

The conclusion to draw from this and related work is not that one can think positive thoughts and throw away one's medications. Optimistic, popular Paul (the fun-loving guy who walked on stilts and played pom-pom pull away as a kid) contracted pneumonia in his early forties. He relied on medical expertise and not just his optimistic nature to recover his health. People traveling on healthy pathways have a whole host of healthy thoughts—and associated feelings and behaviors—that combine to produce a dramatic positive influence on their likelihood of long life.

What It Means for You: Guideposts to Health and Long Life

Douglas Kelley swallowed cyanide more than a decade after seeing the horror of the Nazis up close. His suicide decision appeared sudden and unprovoked. After all, in the intervening years, he'd had a family and built a successful career as a professor, doctor, and researcher. But, from intensive study of the Terman participants, we know that those who committed suicide did not suddenly and erratically fall off the path. Negative thoughts became more and more consuming and started to influence feelings and behaviors.

When the actress Marilyn Monroe was found dead of an overdose of barbiturates at age thirty-six, there was much uncertainty about whether this was an accident, a suicide, or even a murder. Dr. Shneidman was called in to work with the coroner and perform what he called a psychological autopsy. He saw that Marilyn Monroe had come from an unstable family, had faced a difficult childhood, had been impulsive and unreliable, had had many romantic relationships and three marriages, and, as the stress of her career built, had turned to alcohol and prescription drugs. She fit the suicidal pattern, and the coroner ruled her death a probable suicide.

Our studies of catastrophizing, coupled with the explorations of Terman subject suicides by Drs. Tomlinson-Keasey, Shneidman, and others, present a multisided picture of those predisposed to a violent death before age sixty. Such individuals not only faced overly dramatic thoughts but they were inclined to dramatic, precipitous actions. They were not only worried about failures but they were often missing something from childhood—usually a parent's love. They often had headed down a path of alcohol, divorce, or loneliness, but sometimes, as with Douglas Kelley, they had stared into the abyss of a world they could not fathom.

If someone is already far down a self-destructive pathway, the intensive measures needed for detox and sobering up are well-known; they often involve a period of very close monitoring by professionals. But what about someone who has tendencies that could lead in that direction, but who has many strengths as well?

The good news is that catastrophic and related negative thought processes can be changed. The first step is recognizing thoughts for what they are—merely thoughts. This doesn't mean that they are unimportant or hold no power; we have seen dramatic illustrations of their potency in the lives of some of the Terman subjects, for instance. But the power of thoughts can be harnessed, and this is the basic premise behind cognitive therapy.

Cognitive therapy focuses on changing harmful thoughts using techniques such as "thought stopping." When you start to think catastrophic thoughts, you literally say to yourself, "Stop!" This is immediately followed by "thought replacement," which is replacing the negative thoughts with more positive ones. It's actually very difficult to simply not think about something. Try not thinking about a purple penguin. You likely were not thinking of a purple penguin a minute ago, but now that we've brought it to your attention, it's hard to get it out of your head. The best way to banish penguin thoughts is to focus elsewhere. Thought replacement requires the individual who has just stopped a negative thought to replace it with something else—something positive or distracting.

Rationally examining catastrophizing thought patterns and beliefs also proves useful. Most people probably recognize, at least in part, that things aren't *really* as bad as all that, but this nugget of truth gets lost amid all the chaos of perceived calamity. Taking time to thoughtfully evaluate the situation—"What is the worst-case scenario?" or "How likely is it that all of my friends really hate me?"—and to replace inaccurate, catastrophe-oriented thoughts and beliefs with more rational and realistic ones is a worthwhile exercise. Often, writing them down can help. Many recovering catastrophizers benefit from keeping a daily diary, in which they recall the good things that happened today, dismiss the catastrophizing, and write logical plans for tomorrow. But anyone with a troubling, chronic mental health problem should not try to self-diagnose or self-treat. Professional consultations can point one toward the treatments that are most likely to be successful in any particular case.

Again, this may sound simple, but making changes to habitual patterns of thought takes patience, persistence, and determination. Many find that they are too lost in the catastrophizing to do it alone and choose to seek the help of a therapist. Whatever the method, the good news is that catastrophizers do have it in their power to become more realistic, and to learn to laugh it off should an acorn drop on their heads.

· CHAPTER 6 ·

Childhood and School Days

Head Start, Early Finish

Philip, a healthy infant, weighed seven pounds at birth. He was not breast-fed. His toddler years were uneventful. A precocious learner, he began first grade at an unusually young age. How did such early characteristics and experiences affect later health and longevity?

The effects of early life events on later health are puzzling. For example, nutritional problems at a very young age might predispose a child to later heart disease and other adult illnesses, and impaired child-drearing can affect later reactions to stressful challenges; but most children seem unaffected. Severe deficiencies are obviously a problem, but what about the large number of common variations—are these findings about early risks mostly hype, or are they serious factors to worry about?

The Terman children's weight at birth ranged from under six pounds to ten pounds, with the average being about eight pounds. Some were not in good health during their first year while others were quite hearty. Later in childhood, some were judged by Terman and his staff or by physicians to be "below average" in health while others were "very superior." Some had undergone surgeries or had serious accidents during early childhood while others had never been hospitalized. Of course all were doing well enough to be recruited by Terman into his study, and we cannot reach any conclusions here about very ill or traumatized children.

Startlingly, these and many related early health indicators were *not* associated with long life. Generally speaking, a simple early health advantage or disadvantage was not that important to later health trajectories. This does not mean that some such small relations or associations could not be found in a very large study of hundreds of thousands of children. And it certainly is true that significant malnutrition, significant prematurity, or significant exposure to toxins (including prenatal alcohol exposure) can translate into very serious long-term health threats.

However, unless there is brain damage, our research has led us to be skeptical about claims that a single indicator of early health would usually be of lasting significance across the decades for most middle-class people. We found that many aspects of early life do indeed matter, but typically only as part of *general patterns* that build and become more pronounced throughout life.

Breast-Feeding

The typical Terman child was breast-fed for about eight months. But many were not breast-fed at all, and a few were breast-fed until they were three years old.

Perhaps because a newborn is so frail and helpless or perhaps because it's a practice that's entangled with culture and gender wars, breast-feeding often provokes heated debate. Many women worry and struggle as to whether and how long they should breast-feed their babies. In the United States, breast-feeding has taken a place in the pantheon of health behaviors about which to agonize and fret.

There is little doubt that breast-feeding is usually healthy for infants, especially those who are at high risk for illness or are from poor families living in less than optimal conditions. Breast-feeding provides a rich source of nutrients and of protective antibodies, and it can help launch a healthy and continuing mother-child attachment. But how large are the benefits for infants who have access to excellent nutrition without breast-feeding and who are growing up in stable families with sufficient resources to provide a clean, safe environment? Is breast-feeding one of those "must-do" activities that has major long-term effects, or is it one of those behaviors in the long list of things that are helpful but nowhere near essential in promoting a long, healthy life?

The Terman children provided an answer. We knew that studying them could put breast-feeding into the greater context of their lives. We gathered information, originally collected from the parents, on breast-feeding in almost 1,200 of the Terman participants.

Many behaviors and processes associated with breast-feeding, both biological and social, could be relevant to health across the decades. But the simplest and most powerful analysis would ask whether the breast-fed Terman children lived longer and whether they were less likely to die of any particular diseases.

Consistent with other research, we did find that breast-feeding was associated with better infant health. But what about the long term? It turned out that breast-feeding made little difference. There were some indications that the breast-fed males were a little healthier, but no clear patterns really existed. Breast-feeding also seemed, after careful examination, to be unrelated to personality.[33]

All in all, our findings, coupled with the scientific evidence provided by others, suggest that breast-feeding is likely a healthful practice; but in developed areas with good nutrition, it is unlikely to be more than a very minor influence on long-term health and longevity in adulthood.

Early Education

Things got more interesting when we examined early education. Aside from our families, the most important early influences on our paths to health are school and friendships. Infants possess many newly forming abilities and predispositions—some arising from genes and others coming from in-the-womb experiences (such as exposure to hormones) and the early home environment. Some of the Terman infants were active and some were more relaxed; some were shy and some were intrinsically curious about other children. But beyond the influences of these predispositions and our early home lives, it is predominantly in school and among peers that we begin to shape lifelong patterns of competition or cooperation, perseverance or impulsivity, isolation or social integration, and activity or passivity. These patterns, in turn, are linked to later health and longevity.

Before we turn to our examination of the Terman children's early education, pause a moment to reflect on your own early experiences—and answer about yourself some of the same questions the Terman participants' parents answered about them.

SELF-ASSESSMENT: EARLY SCHOOL

Answer the five following questions.

Did you go to preschool?

At what age did you enter regular school (first grade)?

Did you learn to read before starting school?

Was your primary (elementary) school rigid and competitive?

Did you ever skip a grade?

Although all these answers relate to academic progress and achievement, it turns out that it doesn't make sense to add them all together to get an overall score. In fact, as we explored these elements in more detail we found that they were quite different in terms of their relation to mortality risk. So, as we continue, keep your answers in mind.

Head Start?

The Terman children were capable of being good students, and in grade school most of them excelled in literature, composition, history, science, and debate. But they were average or worse in art, shop, and penmanship. That is, Dr. Terman was the first scientist to find real evidence for the common stereotype that all those future doctors, lawyers, and engineers, whatever their other talents, would be sorely lacking in the domain of legible script.

Philip, a precocious but fidgety boy, was enrolled in first grade right at age five. Because they were academically well qualified, a number of the Terman children, like Philip, started school early or skipped a grade.

In contrast, Linda went to kindergarten at age five and started first grade at the normal, traditional age of six, even though she was a very bright and mature girl. Would Linda have been better off if she had gotten a jump on formal schooling? Could something like starting school early or late affect long-term health and longevity?

Traditionally, in America, children attend kindergarten at age five and enter the first grade at age six. (This is not directly dependent on whether they have attended preschool.) Not surprisingly, approximately half the Terman participants entered first grade and started formal schooling at about age six. But a significant number entered school at an earlier age—at age five or even a bit younger than that. Their parents thought they were bright and "ready" for school—they wanted their children to learn as much as possible as soon as possible. Linda's mother, like some other parents, was in no hurry. And she didn't want Linda to be younger than her classmates.

Was Linda's mother on to something or was she being overly cautious? On the one hand, kids who are younger than their classmates can develop low self-esteem and find themselves without adequate grounding for the adolescent scene when they enter middle school. On the other hand, intellectually advanced kids who enter school with peers their own age can become bored and develop behavior problems as a result. So, led by the efforts of Peggy Kern, then a graduate student, we tracked the effects of the starting age on health and longevity across the decades.[34]

We found that those Terman participants who started school at a very early age tended to encounter difficulties throughout their lives. For example, the early-starting boys like Philip were somewhat less likely to grow up to be very well-adjusted adults, and the early-starting girls were more likely to later abuse alcohol.

And surprisingly enough, their age at entering school predicted the subjects' longevity, too. The children who started first grade at age five were at higher risk of dying early, and those who started school on schedule (at age six) lived longer. Just as we had discovered that an element of childhood personality—conscientiousness—was very relevant to health decades later, we now saw that something as seemingly unrelated to health as a school starting age could also tell us something about a person's chances of living a long life.

There was no single ingredient that explained the increased risk for those who started school at a younger-than-average age. Indeed, many of these precocious Terman participants did live long and healthy lives. But it was a mark that something could go very wrong if the children were pushed too far, too fast. Because relating to classmates is so important for children, an out-of-sync start can launch some of them down some erratic paths. We concluded that parents should not enroll their kids at age five in an attempt to give them an advantage. Getting an early start—jumping ahead of one's peers—is a dead-end myth.

What About Skipping Ahead?

Linda was not an early starter, but she was an easy starter. She did well in all of her classes, even penmanship. She had many friends, and her teacher observed that she was unselfish and had a level of common sense that was "above average." She enjoyed her dolls and playing hopscotch. Thus, she was a "traditionalist" both in school age and activities. Linda also liked to study—everything seemed easy for her to learn. Linda in fact accelerated in her third-grade year, completing two grades in that same year and skipping on to fifth grade. Was that a good idea?

Because the Terman children entered school at different ages, and because some skipped or repeated grades, they had very different grade school experiences. At the end of eighth grade, some students were the same age as their classmates, while others were older or younger. We wondered if the onset of adolescence was the key turning point. But it wasn't: age match with peers as a teenager was not significantly related to mortality risk; it was age at school *entry* that made the difference. Linda, for example, remained popular and well-adjusted, continued to do well in school, and appeared to be no worse off for having sprinted through her third- and fourth-grade years.

Playtime

So maybe the problem with early school entry was pushy parents, relentlessly pressing their preschoolers to get ahead. To check, we considered that perhaps what really mattered was the age at which the child learned to read. In fact, about a third of the children learned to read before first grade, especially those who had more preschool instruction and whose parents were better educated and of a higher occupational status. Did it matter? To long life, no. Being a very early reader was associated with somewhat poorer mental adjustment later in life, but the age at which the child started reading was not related to lifelong mortality risk. Being bright and precocious was not the problem. The problem was starting formal schooling too young.

To understand these findings, let's consider Philip. A bright boy, even compared to other Terman subjects, Philip was a front-runner in many areas. He moved from a bottle to solid food at an earlier age than most infants, his teeth came in early, and he walked and talked earlier than other children. Even his worries seemed adultlike. He was energetic, outgoing, and clearly very smart, so it's not surprising that his mother wanted to channel this energy and brilliance into something more constructive than taking apart his toys and racing pell-mell up and down the stairs. She may have also hoped that the structured environment of the classroom would help make Philip more responsible and diligent—he was friendly and popular but not very conscientious or persistent.

Unfortunately her plan didn't work. By entering formal instruction at a very early age, Philip lost the unstructured playtime that psychologists know to be so important to healthy development. Philip's performance in school was competent but uneven. In some areas (those that interested him) his teacher rated him as "very superior" but in subjects he cared less about, he was only average. His attitude in his early school years suggested that he was "anxious to outdistance others, to progress or excel" but despite this, he exhibited little follow-through in areas that failed to draw his attention. He was generally well liked by his peers, and not often teased, but his teacher remarked that he tended to "seek attention by behavior." Accelerating the pace of life for this precocious and anxiety-prone child reinforced unhealthy levels of stress.

We know now (although it was not understood then) that the brains of children, and even teenagers, are still developing. Philip's problems with impulse control and focus were not likely to be helped by a competitive classroom environment. And, being one of the youngest in the class, he probably felt the need to prove himself.

Higher Education

Education is a great predictor of future income in our society—college graduates earn much more than high school graduates, and those with graduate degrees tend to do better than those without. There is also very good evidence from various studies that socioeconomic status is relevant to health. But this doesn't necessarily mean that getting more education will make you live longer.

It is usually difficult to separate influences of education from influences of intelligence—smarter individuals generally go further in school, are healthier, understand more about health, and live longer. So we thought it would be important to examine education and its effect among the Terman participants, all of whom were smart. Did the best-educated subjects live the longest?

Pretty much all of the Terman participants attended at least some high school and about two-thirds graduated from college, with many of them going on to get graduate degrees. That left many others who did not go to or finish college. In fact fifty-three men flunked out! They were all smart but lots of things in life mattered more than intelligence in determining who would become highly educated. Fewer than a third of those in college graduated with honors—given how intelligent they were, it seemed many did not try very hard.

We were surprised to find that level of education by itself was not a very good predictor of later health and longevity. The better-educated Terman subjects did tend to be healthier and live a little longer, but this was not an important factor compared to other personal and social predictors of health and long life that often went along with success in school. The better educated were more productive as they aged—they were more successful in their careers and more likely to continue to work, grow personally, be creative, and "do" things. But this was not primarily because of their education. Instead it was because they were the kind of persistent people who were better able and better motivated to navigate life's personal and social challenges.

Those participants who went on to be better educated, more successful, and healthier had parents who were better educated and more successful themselves. Their parents valued the accomplishments of the highly proficient members of society. Such high expectations and supportive social environments then combined with inherent characteristics of certain children and helped push them down healthier pathways of life.

What It Means for You: Guideposts to Health and Long Life

By the time of his death in 1956, Dr. Terman and his study had discredited the stereotype of child prodigy as nerd, geek, or weirdo. Over 95 percent of these bright children were still participating in the study, and the majority continued to flourish and achieve in multiple domains. But despite their natural abilities, these people differed in their personalities, their perseverance, and the deeper education they achieved. Those who thrived in their schooling from childhood on and managed to apply their skills to interpersonal and social spheres did well not only in life but in health. Except they never did manage to polish their awful handwriting.

These days there is increasing attention to early life experiences and later life health. This is both good and bad. The good side is that health professionals are starting to recognize that many diseases of middle age have some very early origins. The bad side is that these risks are often seen as much more threatening and much less changeable than they really are. We have found that a number of important health-relevant patterns are usually launched in childhood and youth but also that these patterns *can be altered and improved.* In the coming chapters we'll explore some of these in detail—patterns of marriage and divorce, good and bad exercise, career successes and failures, religions and congregations, and more.

A few aspects of school days had clear links to health and longevity: starting formal schooling at a very early age turned out not to be a very good idea for most. Many early starters strayed off the paths that would have led them to become well-adjusted adults who took care of their health. They were less likely to live a long life.

Nevertheless, not everyone was negatively affected by an accelerated academic schedule. Take, for example, Lee Cronbach. A publicly identified Terman participant, Cronbach later became well-known in the fields of educational psychology and psychological testing. When he was only four years old, Cronbach was overheard calculating the unit price of potatoes and comparing the value to be found at one market versus another.[35] His mother was anxious for him to excel and enrolled him in second grade soon after his fifth birthday. At eighteen, when most boys were graduating from high school, Lee was graduating from college. Importantly, he went on to marry, have children, and build an illustrious career. He lived to be eighty-five years old. As we later found when we delved deeply into the lives, marriages, and careers of the Terman men and women, those who faced stresses early in life but who bounced back by young adulthood were able to overcome early threats to their later health.

What if you started first grade early, had a rough time in school, were kind of sickly, and never made it to graduate school? Is it time to see your doctor? Not necessarily. Many other factors turned out to be much more important on the paths to long life.

CHAPTER 7

Parental Divorce

Some Were Resilient

Donna's parents divorced in 1924, when she was thirteen years old. Donna had enjoyed her family life, and the split was hard on her. Although she went on to a successful career in advertising, she never fully recovered from the family breakup. It seemed eventually to affect her health, and Donna died in 1970, at the relatively young age of fifty-nine. We wondered if a story similar to Donna's played out among other Terman children, and if so, what long-term paths might characterize Donna and the others. How could something that happened at age thirteen lead to death at age fifty-nine?

It is well established that divorce of parents can be harmful for the children, at least in the short term. But what about in the long term, across the decades? Could the child's experience of divorce be related to mortality risk many years in the future?

Health researchers haven't much considered or investigated whether divorce of one's parents and related family problems in childhood would create a significant risk for later heart disease, cancer, and other health threats. Divorce of one's parents is not a biological risk factor like having high cholesterol in one's blood. Physicians generally don't ask their adult patients about it, although pediatricians may worry about short-term threats in the teenage years.

It is very rare to be able to follow children from divorced families for many decades into the future. Little was known about long-term health effects until we began our studies of the Terman participants.

As with Donna, Patricia's parents had divorced when she was young—only ten years old. James and fidgety Philip, too, came from families with dissolved marriages. Would outcomes be similar for all of them or would there be striking differences? When they grew up, would the divorce be relevant to their own marriages as well?

Parental Divorce and Longevity

Any parent contemplating divorce worries about how the change will affect their children. To gauge those effects on the Terman children, we looked at two events that shatter families—death and divorce. More than a third of the Terman children faced one of these circumstances before they reached age twenty-one.

The death of a parent is certainly traumatic for children, which is why communities and religious groups have developed various rituals and ways of cushioning the blow for survivors. Would the death of a parent have negative long-term effects? We were surprised to find that although the death of a parent during one's childhood was usually difficult, it had no measurable impact on life-span mortality risk. The children adapted and moved on with their lives.

That was the end of the good news. Although losing one's parent to divorce might seem better than losing a parent through death, we found the opposite. The long-term health effects of parental divorce were often devastating—it was indeed a risky circumstance that changed the pathways of many of the young Terman participants. Children from divorced families died almost five years earlier on average than children from intact families. Parental divorce, not parental death, was the risk. In fact, parental divorce during childhood was the single strongest social predictor of early death, many years into the future.[36]

When her parents split up, Donna and her brother stayed with their mother. Donna continued to go to the same school and occasionally the same Lutheran church. Her mother found a position as an office worker, and there seemed to be little overt disruption in Donna's life. Around the time when Donna was learning to drive, her mother married again. Soon thereafter, Donna moved on to college, a career, and a family of her own.

Philip's parents also divorced when he was thirteen. He was close to both his mother and father and later reported that he rarely argued with either of them. By his own account, their split was a significant event in his life. He, too, remained with his mother after the separation, but, unlike Donna's mother, Philip's mother struggled to make ends meet. Philip's tendencies toward anxiety and worry had been exacerbated by the stress of his parents' divorce and subsequent lack of stability, and so he must have felt some relief as he joined the armed forces and took more direct control over his life. The structure and routine of military life seemed to suit him, and he spent a number of years in the service. Nevertheless, in 1950 he reported to Dr. Terman that he felt he hadn't lived up to his potential, and he expressed less than complete satisfaction with his work. Philip, too, married and started a family before joining the overseas war effort in 1941. He died of a heart attack in 1974. He was sixty-four years old.

Living Through Divorce, Dying Young

Both Donna and Philip died at a relatively young age. What was linking the experience of parental divorce to higher mortality risk?[37] Given that both we and other researchers had found that the death of a parent is usually not a long-term health threat, we thought it must be something about the breakup of the family, perhaps the strife and distress.

Although it may seem counterintuitive, the first thing we needed to do was to see if the child was the problem. We knew that unconscientious children and those who had certain other characteristics in the "untamed" direction (i.e., impulsiveness and moodiness) were less likely to live long lives. So perhaps it was Donna's unconscientious acting-out that was both driving her parents to divorce and then lead-ing to her own early demise. Or, to put it bluntly, it would be Donna's fault not her parents' fault. If true, this would be important to know, because it would mean that parental divorce was not playing a causal role in the later premature deaths of these Terman children.

We found that the effects of childhood personality and the effects of experiencing the parents' divorce were not related to each other. Each was an independent health risk factor. The problem emerging from stressed families was not in fact coming from the children. In addition, although serious illness or serious disability of a child can cause strain on a marriage, that was not what was going on in Dr. Ter-man's sample of 1,528 bright and generally healthy children.

Marriage and divorce have different meanings for males and fe-males, so we separated our statistical analyses by sex. With then–graduate student Joan Tucker leading the way, we pulled out the death certificates we had gathered and checked the causes of death. Things were indeed different for boys than for girls. We found that the men who, as children, had faced parental divorce were especially likely to die of accidents or violence, suggesting they grew up to be more reck-less. But both the men and the women who had faced parental divorce were also more likely to die sooner from all other causes, including cancer and heart attack and stroke. In other words, parental divorce was a general and powerful risk factor, especially relevant to death from injury but also relevant to death from disease.

Divorce can drastically alter a family's finances, and so we won-dered if financial hardship was promoting long-term risks following a divorce. Although the Terman participants were mostly middle class, there were variations in socioeconomic status (measured by a combi-nation of income, occupation, and education). As a whole, divorce tended to lower the children's standard of living, but individual dif-ferences among families were evident. Donna's mother was able to become self-sufficient rather quickly, while Philip's mother struggled financially until he left home. Looking at the group as a whole, we dis-covered that a plunge in childhood socioeconomic status did make a difference for some of these children of divorce, especially for the girls.

But surprisingly, other factors were much more important. Discovering the true pathways to long life revealed that a solution to this threat would not be primarily economic.

The Real Problem with Parental Divorce

How did the children of divorce differ from the children from intact families once they had all grown up? We wondered if the two groups had achieved different educational levels. Indeed, one difference was that both boys and girls from divorced homes tended to end their education earlier than those from intact families—many were discouraged and had fallen off the track of upward mobility. This handicap affected not only their future income but also their overall career accomplishments. The gap made a difference for boys, helping to explain part of their increased mortality risk. Men were expected, during the Terman era, to be the head of the family. Less accomplishment limited their ability to do this effectively, decreasing their status in adulthood and increasing their stress-filled behavior patterns and their risk of dying. The disadvantage was less important for the Terman girls, probably because women during this time period weren't expected to focus as much on work and other activities outside the home.

Heavy drinking and smoking are, of course, significant health risks, and children of divorce, it turned out, engaged in these practices more than Terman subjects from intact homes. This was especially true of smoking. Only a quarter of the men from divorced families never smoked, compared to over a third of the men from intact families. For women, the differences were especially dramatic: women from intact families were more than twice as likely to avoid smoking as those whose parents divorced. And women from divorced families were more than twice as likely to be heavy smokers. Donna, something of a tomboy and rebel, began smoking immediately upon entering college and kept it up for the rest of her life.

Taking into account how much women from divorced families smoked is very useful in explaining their greater mortality risk—the early shattering of their family security predicted a more dangerous lifestyle over the long term. Whereas other researchers had confirmed increased short-term risk for the children of divorce, our findings pointed to the very real long-term impacts. The findings are also consistent with epidemiological studies showing that offspring of divorced parents have increased cancer risks, especially cancers related to tobacco, alcohol, and sexual promiscuity.[38] But even smoking and drinking were not the major key to understanding the increased risk of dying for people like Donna and Philip.

History Repeats Itself

Those who had lived through a divorce as children were much more likely to get divorced themselves. And these later disruptions in their relationships placed them at significantly greater mortality risk. This pattern was especially damaging for men. Uncovering this link was one of our most important findings.

The pattern played out for both Philip and Donna. Donna, who managed to balance a successful career with mothering two active sons, wasn't able to hold her own marriage together. The boys stayed with her, and, like her own divorced mother, Donna was able to provide a stable transition and financial security for them as they grew. But with her unstable childhood, her divorce, and the demands of her job, she was unable to maintain a close circle of friends. She couldn't quit smoking, couldn't maintain her weight, and died of lung cancer.

Philip's marriage also ended in divorce, soon after his return from the Pacific in World War II. It's hard to say to what extent his divorce stemmed from the separation and stresses of war versus from his previous experience with the marital discord of his parents. What we do know is that, whatever the reasons behind it, divorce was a major health risk factor for him and for many of the Terman participants. One key problem was that those who had experienced parental divorce reported fewer group memberships and poorer community relations when they themselves became adults. We will return to this important topic later in this book when we discuss the health and long life significance of stable relationships and certain kinds of social ties.

Rising from the Ashes?

Despite the very real risks associated with parental divorce, there were many Terman children, such as Patricia and James, who experienced the divorce of their parents and went on to live long lives. It is probably an exaggeration to say that some of the Terman participants were like a phoenix rising, but what enabled some of these individuals to manage, and even thrive, in the face of adversity? Most studies would be unable to follow up and see what was helpful. But due to the tremendous efforts of Terman and his colleagues and successors, we could undertake just such a study.

Patricia and James both bounced back—they lived long lives despite having faced a significant risk factor during their childhoods. Their own marriages—James to Irene after a whirlwind courtship, and Patricia to Charles after a cautious and lengthy engagement—were fulfilling, and almost surely played an important role in promoting their longevity.

Both James, the tactful, charismatic one, and prudent Patricia reported that they had many interests in common with their spouses and viewed their marriages as decidedly above average. They also clearly said that if they were to do it all over again, they would choose the same person to marry. (This marital match is not insignificant, as we will see when we examine marriage in detail.) Neither Patricia nor James smoked, neither had been sorely disadvantaged by the parental divorce in terms of their socioeconomic status, and both had completed a good education. Patricia had gone straight through a four-year college and almost immediately started working as a claims adjuster for a well-respected insurance company. James, despite a few setbacks, had eventually completed a four-year degree. All of these were relevant to their longevity. Yet we sensed there might be something else in play.

From looking at the Terman subjects' pathways to long life, we surmised that something about their childhood family environments must be somehow relevant to their health over the long haul. Fortunately, Dr. Terman, the test-everything empiricist, had collected information about whether they were psychologically attached to their parents, how much admiration and affection they felt for each parent, and how helpful their parents had been to them. We put such questions together as a means of measuring positive family environment. It turned out that positive family attributes were more likely to be found in the intact families than in the parental divorce group. This was not surprising. What was surprising was what mattered to those who faced parental divorce.

A good deal of research by others points to the potential long-term problems associated with what are sometimes called risky families—homes that lack nurturance and are instead characterized by conflict.[39] We wondered if children coming from such at-risk environments—parental divorce *and* lack of positive family feelings—might be especially vulnerable, and conversely whether more positive family environments might serve as a kind of buffer for those facing a parental split.

Positive family characteristics were not at all important in the way we had expected. For the boys in the parental divorce group, positive family feelings were *harmful* to the boys—such boys lived shorter lives.[40] It was especially traumatic to have a seemingly positive, functional home torn apart. In contrast, for cases where the family was clearly troubled, the outcome proved to be something of a relief.[41] This finding is in line with the sometimes-heard recommendation that staying married for the sake of the children is usually not a good idea. We would clarify this recommendation, however, by adding that staying married for the sake of the children is usually not a good idea *if the family environment is a distressed and unhappy one.*

For girls, this aspect of family life was not relevant to their later longevity. To be honest, we don't know why. But as we will see later on, different things were often more relevant to the health and longevity of the Terman men than to the Terman women.

The Power of Bouncing Back

Beyond having healthy marriages and avoiding cigarettes and other dangerous habits, Patricia and James—the survivors—had something else in common. In 1950 they and other resilient subjects reported deep satisfaction and interest in their vocations and felt they had lived up to their intellectual abilities. Contrast this with Philip, who, you will recall, reported that he hadn't lived up to his potential and that although he wasn't totally discontented with his career, neither did he find it wholly satisfying.

This sense of being satisfied with one's life and achievement was very relevant to resilience. The Terman participants (especially men) who found a sense of personal satisfaction and accomplishment by midlife were buffered against the ill effects of their childhood traumas. This may sound commonsensical. The startling twist, however, was that this sense of satisfaction predicted longer life spans *only* for those whose parents had divorced. Although the rest—those whose parents had stayed married—surely felt good about their accomplishments (or bad about their lack of accomplishments), that sense of satisfaction did not at all affect their mortality risk. This protective strength—this added health-relevant maturity—emerged in the presence of the challenge of parental divorce. Individuals who were able to call up resilience in order to overcome hardship had longer lives.

So there really is something to say for becoming stronger by overcoming adversity. An interesting side note is that most studies of stress and resilience could never uncover such a finding, because they would not be able to make the necessary comparisons. Most studies of individuals facing trauma or stress would endeavor to see who is resilient, but would not include individuals who were *not* facing trauma, divorce, or stress. As such, they wouldn't be able to tell us whether protective patterns are generally helpful in facing life's challenges or just valuable to those facing a special or intense stress.

Resilient Temperaments

Was there perhaps also something about the temperaments or personalities of certain Terman subjects that helped make them resilient? Did some children have internal qualities that helped them withstand the pummeling of a troubled home? These aren't novel questions: other researchers have found evidence that individual factors, some of which are genetic, contribute to the negative outcomes associated with experiencing parental divorce.[42] That is, children with difficult temperaments seem to have more trouble adapting to change and also tend to elicit negative emotions and behaviors from others, whereas those with easy temperaments garner less negativity and cope better with what they do experience.

We therefore looked to see whether the Terman subjects' personalities could be moderating the effect—influencing their experience of, and reaction to, the dissolution of their parents' marriage in a way that was relevant to their life-span mortality risk. Were some just born resilient? Not at all. Just as their personalities were not causing their parents' breakups, those who matured and became satisfied with their lives and their work did so because they found some strength of character, not because of their temperament or personality. Resilience was cultivated throughout their early adult years; they grappled with the challenge, overcame it, and went on to live long lives.

Divorce Rates Today

In American society today, about half of all first marriages end in divorce; the rates of divorce for second and third marriages climb even higher. This rate is higher than it was when the Terman subjects were children. For those whose parents divorced, there was more stigma and more uncertainty, whereas today's children of divorce are rarely stigmatized and likely have friends in the same situation. In some communities, complete and stable family units in fact seem to be aberrations. Yet even when divorce is the norm, research studies today still find that it is traumatic and harmful to children—in terms of their mental health, in terms of their potential for drug abuse, and more. In this sense, contemporary youth is not so different from the Terman kids—leading us to believe, from our reading of the evidence, that family breakups today are not just an economic threat and a threat to the short-term well-being of children and teenagers, but they can also be a threat to long-term health and well-being.

The good news, on the other hand, is that the risk from parental divorce is not inevitable. Children like Patricia and James, who are not plunged into poverty and who do not turn to harmful habits such as smoking to help them cope or fit in with peers, can dodge the risk. In particular, those who are later able to establish a stable and meaningful relationship with a partner and who find passion and fulfillment in their work can overcome the legacy of divorce. As we shall see in later chapters, the Terman participants showed us the paths on which emotional healing can be found and how old wounds can be put to rest.

SELF-ASSESSMENT: LIFE SATISFACTION

Answer each of the following questions as honestly as you can.

1. Which of the following best describes your feeling about your present vocation?

    Deep satisfaction and interest in my work _____(5)

    Fairly content _____(4)

    No serious discontent, but don't find it especially interesting or satisfying _____(3)

    Discontented but will probably stick it out _____(2)

    Strongly dislike and hope to change _____(1)

2. On the whole, how well do you think you have lived up to your intellectual abilities and potential? (Don't limit your answer to economic or vocational success only.)

    Fully—have been reaching my potential _____(5)

    Reasonably well _____(4)

    Considerably short of it _____(3)

    Consider my accomplishments weak _____(2)

    Pretty much a failure _____(1)

3. Which of the following best describes your satisfaction with your everyday life?

    Love every aspect of it _____(5)

    Am satisfied and content with most aspects _____(4)

    It has a balance of good and bad _____(3)

    I have little to look forward to each day _____(2)

    Dislike most aspects of it _____(1)

4. In all, do you feel you are where you should be in fulfilling the plans and dreams you have for your life?

    Absolutely _____(5)

    For the most part, yes _____(4)

    In some areas yes, but not in others _____(3)

    For the most part, no _____(2)

    Not at all _____(1)

5. If you were to start your life over again, which would be your approach?

    I wouldn't change a thing _____(5)

    I would change very little _____(4)

    I would make some moderate changes _____(3)

    I would probably change many things _____(2)

    I would change almost all of it _____(1)

6. Which of the following best describes your contentment with your social life?

    Completely content, it's just right _____(5)

    Quite content, I'm seldom lonely or overwhelmed with too many activities _____(4)

    Neither content nor otherwise _____(3)

    Quite discontented, I'm often too lonely or am overwhelmed with excessive socializing _____(2)

    Completely discontented, it's not at all what I would prefer _____(1)

Scoring: Each of the questions has five options, and they are listed in descending order with regard to satisfaction—that is, the first response for each question indicates the greatest satisfaction and receives a score of 5 and the last response indicates the least and receives a score of 1. Add up the total. Your score should fall between 6 and 30. If you scored at least 20 you are in the upper quartile (25 percent) in terms of being satisfied with your life. The lower quartile scores around 15 and below.

For those who endured the trauma of their parents' divorce, having gained a sense of competence, maturity, and satisfaction in adulthood are very good signs that one has bounced back from the stress one bore. For those who faced parental divorce and have a low score on satisfaction with life and accomplishments, this combination could be a warning sign of health risks to come. But it is only one sign, and it should be considered in the context of the other risk factors we'll be describing.

What It Means for You: Guideposts to Health and Long Life

Parents sometimes wisecrack that they sleep in separate bedrooms, keep separate checking accounts, and take separate vacations—anything to keep their marriage together. But divorce is no joke to the children. Our studies revealed that the stress of family discord and especially parental divorce is important not only in the short term but to a person's entire life path. Fortunately, we also uncovered a little-explored route off the main highway—a road toward resilience.

We found no long-term health effects coming from the early death of a parent. Instead, it was the conflict and stress of a disintegrating family that proved to be problematic. The children who lived through ongoing clashes and those who were shocked by a seemingly sudden split took things especially badly. Many turned to unhealthy behaviors like smoking and headed down unhealthy pathways in which they did not reach their educational and career potential.

That said, the Terman participants who were able, despite the dysfunctional patterns they observed in childhood, to establish themselves in good marriages of their own were much better off in terms of their future health and longevity than were those who followed the template their parents modeled for them. Most important, achieving a sense of satisfaction and a sense of accomplishment by young adulthood had a valuable buffering effect. These mature individuals had strengthened themselves and embarked on the path to long life.

Patricia and James were both able to develop these resilient patterns, perhaps learning from their parents' mistakes and resolving to do differently in their own lives. Sure, they did the right things in other ways, too, by trying to avoid unhealthy habits and by persevering toward their educational and career goals. But through their deeper patterns of living—toward satisfaction in life and good marriages—they were able to thrive despite the challenges they encountered. In other words, having one's parents split up does not necessarily mean increased health risks for an individual, but rather it may make working at one's own situation particularly important, with correspondingly greater benefits.

CHAPTER 8

Running for Their Lives

Jocks vs. Nerds

A ncel Keys was a very active man. One of the publicly identified Terman study participants, Keys became world famous in public health. Most people know of his work even if they do not know his name. Ancel Keys was also one of the longest living Terman subjects. As a toddler, he survived the San Francisco earthquake of 1906. After a very long and eventful life, he died in 2004, at the age of one hundred.

As a young man Ancel worked first in a lumber camp, and then as a gold miner, a ship's oiler, a manager, and a scientist. After receiving his doctorate in biology, he continued to travel ardently, even going to the Chilean Andes to study the physiological effects of high altitudes. Keys was the nephew of actor Lon Chaney but that was not his claim to fame. He is notable for his work on fats, cholesterol, and heart disease.

During the Second World War, Dr. Keys, well-regarded for his expertise in human physiology, was asked by the U.S. government to develop a food bundle or ration pack that was nutritious and compact and could be readily used by combat troops. His package—of dry biscuits, protein from peanuts or sausage, and chocolate—was modified in a number of ways and became the famous K ration. Keys liked to claim that the K ration was named after him, but there is evidence that the *K* was simply chosen by the bureaucracy as a distinct letter of the alphabet.[43]

After the war Dr. Keys, noting the significant incidence of heart disease in western societies, began studying its causes. He is the person most responsible for the idea that a high-fat diet leads to high cholesterol and heart disease. Like Ignaz Semmelweis, the nineteenth-century doctor who blamed the "child-bed fever" of mothers in labor on germs but was met with scorn and disbelief, Keys also faced skepticism and personal attacks. Yet he persisted, eventually recommending the so-called Mediterranean diet that emphasizes fruits, vegetables, beans, cereals, nuts, and unsaturated fat. Although his idea about dietary fat and heart disease remained quite controversial for many years (and still has significant critics arguing over the details), it became one of the most important topics in cardiology and public health.

In 1961 Keys was featured on the cover of *Time* magazine. He made it clear that he thought that Americans were eating too much. Yet today, half a century later, Americans eat even more, and obesity rates are much, much higher. He also made it clear that Americans were eating too much saturated fat. Keys himself did not avoid red meat; he just limited how much of it he ate each week. Today everyone has heard about cholesterol, many are obsessed with it, and countless individuals have switched to unbalanced, unproven diets. Cardiovascular disease remains the leading cause of death. Simply providing information ("You eat too much") and lists of recommendations ("Eat less fat") to the public turned out to be an ineffective public health strategy.

Ancel Keys strongly believed that physical activity was essential to good health—and he continued his vigorous activities throughout his life. But he preferred staying active in the service of interests, chores, and hobbies, such as travel or gardening. He was not a proponent of marathons or bodybuilding contests. He stayed trim and active not because of any secret, special exercise regimen but because of life-long patterns that he developed. We decided to focus intensively on figuring out the physical activity patterns of all the Terman subjects. Did the active children become active adults? What was the personality of those who stayed active? Was physical activity very important to health and long life?

The Exercise Thermometer

Because we have thousands of pieces of information that were collected across eight decades on over 1,500 Terman participants, we sit looking at almost 10 million facts and pieces of data. What kinds of health-relevant behavior could be measured throughout life? How could we best assess physical activity?

These days, exercise researchers like to use a measure called the metabolic equivalent, or MET. One MET describes your calorie consumption when you are at rest—you are alive but not doing anything. Serious jogging is 8 METs. Hard running is 18 METs. Throughout their lives, the Terman participants were asked about their hobbies, sports, and activity levels. So we are able to construct good estimates throughout the decades that are comparable to those that modern-day researchers use.

Some Terman participants liked reading, movies, and board games. Others preferred gardening, boating, woodwork, photography, or travel. Still others chose team sports, handball, hunting, hiking, or skiing. By assigning a MET value to each activity, Peggy Kern and the rest of our team were able to compute the average physical activity of each Terman participant. Not only that, but we could examine how activity levels changed across the decades, and thus be better able to make sensible, valid prescriptions for optimally active lifestyles.[44]

Varieties of Fitness

It is common to hear advice to exercise more in order to stay healthy. In other words, make up your mind to be healthy and get out on the tennis or basketball court. On New Year's Day, many resolve to spend more time in the gym; by March, well, the gym has empty slots. This exercise advice comes from the common observation that those who are physically active are generally healthier. But this advice ignores your individual personality and your past history of activity or inactivity. What if you are already a tennis player? Should you then add triathlon competitions? What if you used to play a lot of tennis but now prefer strolling from store to store, shopping? Are you more or less healthy than a couch potato?

A different way to think about physical activity is to put people into categories. Some seem very active—the jocks—and some seem to have little interest in active recreation—the nerds. If this approach is more valid in capturing reality, then there is little point in berating the nerds—they simply are not going to develop and sustain a very active life. But if the categories are loose ones, perhaps some nerds might be induced to increase their physical activity. And jocks could be encouraged to maintain their activities over many years, rather than fading with age (as many do).

On the occasion of his seventieth birthday, Mark Twain said:

I have never taken any exercise, except sleeping and resting, and I never intend to take any. Exercise is loathsome. And it cannot be any benefit when you are tired; and I was always tired.[45]

But it is what Twain said next that especially piqued our research interest:

I desire now to repeat and emphasize that maxim: We can't reach old age by another man's road. My habits protect my life, but they would assassinate you.

We knew there were huge differences in the Terman subjects' personalities, and so we decided to investigate all of these possibilities. Are some individuals basically more active than others? Do their activity levels persist over time? What is relevant to health and long life?

Active Children, Active Adults?

In 1922, when they were about eleven years old, the Terman children were evaluated in terms of their physical activity levels. For example, their parents indicated on a five-point scale how much the child enjoyed playing games that required lots of exercise. They also rated the children's energy levels and described their children's hobbies. Then Dr. Terman asked about a wide variety of activities, ranging from flying kites and hiking, which were popular among the boys, to dancing and playing jackstones (now called jacks), popular among the girls.

In adulthood, the Terman subjects provided all sorts of information about their hobbies, and as noted, we coded each of these as to how active each was. Even in their old age, the participants shared enough information for us to evaluate whether they were participating in sports, active in hobbies like gardening, engaging in exercise programs, and so on. No study had ever before been able to look in such detail at physical activity across the life span, from childhood through aging and until death.

The initial results were amazing. There was definitely some consistency in physical activity levels throughout life. Many people became more active over time and many became less active, but overall there was stability. For example, the parent ratings of their child's energy and activities when he or she was around age eleven or twelve were predictive of activity levels of their hobbies decades later.[46]

John, who became the shy physicist and lived a long life, loved to bicycle and swim at age twelve and loved skiing in the Sierras at age forty-one. Linda was active in both childhood and adulthood; a sociable child, her favorite pastimes in 1922, in addition to playing with dolls, included hopscotch, bouncing a ball, and other outdoor games. Later on she reported dancing, gardening, and tennis as her favorite hobbies and gravitated toward pursuits involving physical exertion.

Some of the patterns, like Donna's, were much more sedentary. As a preteen Donna preferred to spend time playing chess or working on her collections—she had a large assemblage of railroad artifacts, as well as many marbles and arrowheads. Only sometimes did she play actively outside. In high school she became quite a sports enthusiast—but only as a spectator! And in 1950 she listed watching sports and playing cards among her favorite leisure activities.

When designing treatments for a patient with tension headaches or for those who really need to lose weight, doctors surely ask about the duration of the person's condition and for information about what activities and events make it better or worse. Were you overweight as a child? Do you regain lost weight? When did your headaches start? Are your headaches worse in the summer? Yet when on the topic of physical fitness, the doctor will rarely delve into childhood activities, ask about college sports, or look for other such patterns. Instead, the advice will usually be, "You should increase your exercise, maybe take up running or join an exercise class." But there is a better way to proceed.

Fitness levels, it appears, are more personal than the general "exercise is good for you" mantra might suggest. All in all, the findings told us that it makes no sense to rely on generalizations—individuals, we found, are on their own activity paths. The edict to exercise rigorously needs to be altered and tailored person to person.

METs (Activity) Across the Decades

The metabolic equivalents—the physical activity levels—varied quite a lot among the Terman subjects and across the decades. The men were, on average, more active than the women, but there were many individual patterns. Some were active as children and stayed very active, while others who crocheted and played croquet as children grew up to sew, play cards, and socialize as adults.

There was a decline in physical activity for most of the Terman participants after the teenage years and college, but it then seemed to stabilize and level off. Unsurprisingly, activity gradually decreased as the participants aged but often did not diminish substantially until old age. Even here, it was somewhat different for each individual. By

1972 Linda was no longer playing tennis, but she did continue to garden. John, however, was still quite physically active—now in his sixties he was still skiing. He described his energy and vitality by noting: "Vigorous; have considerable endurance."

Over the next decade plus, the same trends continued for these two—Linda stayed actively engaged in life (she said that she had enough energy for a "full program of activities"), but her actual physical activity continued to decline slowly and by 1986 she worked in her garden only occasionally, spending most of her free time meeting with social groups and visiting informally with friends and neighbors. She also listed a daily nap among her activities. John was unusual—his decrease in physical activity was hardly even noticeable. At each assessment he listed a number of activities, and by 1986 John was still skiing occasionally, walking or hiking frequently, and even cutting his own firewood.

The children who were more sociable—that is, who were popular, often a leader, liked being in large groups, and liked playing with others—generally grew up to be more active adults. This social tendency worked to help them stay involved in sports. But over long periods of years, they tended to decrease their activity levels, so that by the time they reached their sixties, they were no longer more active than their less sociable counterparts. This was especially true for the men in the group, who may have gradually lost contact with organized sports.

The children who were energetic grew up to be adults who were energetic. They were also happier and better adjusted, based on midlife assessments. But for most, by the time they reached their sixties, they, too, looked pretty much like the other Terman participants—no longer significantly more active. Again the pressures of everyday life had limited and homogenized the hobbies. The skiers had become golfers, and the swimmers had become shoppers.

What about the sensitive worriers, those who were lacking in self-confidence? Those who were more neurotic were less likely to be physically active as children and even more unlikely to remain physically active as adults. They tended to avoid rigorous activity, both as children and as adults. They would not go tearing down the ski slopes no matter how many messages they received to get out and exercise.

There were exceptions. James, who was sensitive to the reactions of others in childhood and certainly qualified as one of the more neurotic Terman subjects in adulthood, nonetheless was fairly active throughout his life. Although he didn't take many risks, he did get out and do things. In high school he was on the track team, and he channeled his love for plays into an active role doing stage work and lighting, which can be quite strenuous. As an adult he remained active. His involvement with plays eventually extended only to watching them, but he did continue with the woodworking he had learned in high school. He also enjoyed hiking, birdwatching, and swimming. And, in late life, he was one who specifically noted that he was making an effort to exercise and eat healthfully.

Physical Activity and Long Life

When we looked across the decades, we found that being active in middle age was most important to health and longevity. Being a childhood jock did not lead to long life if you were one of those who quit sports and slowed down a lot as you aged. On the other hand, being inactive in childhood was not a problem if you became more active as you aged. Those who were active in youth and stayed active tended to live very long lives, as was the case with James. Those who were inactive in youth and became more active often did almost as well in terms of life span, and sometimes equally well.

Those who were active were more likely to stay active, but if they did not, their risk of dying increased substantially. The good news for those seeking long life is that physical activity levels improved for many folks over time. Those sedentary desk jockeys who managed to bring out their inner athlete and move their bodies were able to catch up to or even surpass the health of their more naturally active peers.

The Truth About Jogging

There is a dirty little secret known to health professionals that they do not usually much talk about. Let's assume that you follow the recommendations of a health authority and get out there most days to go jogging, even though you would much rather be doing something else. Say you get ready, warm up, jog, and cool down for about an hour a day, which is a modest regimen.

Over a year, you will spend about 360 hours doing this, and during 40 years (say, from age twenty-one to age sixty-one), you will spend about 14,400 hours. Assuming that most of us are awake for about 16 hours a day, this means that you would be spending the equivalent of about 900 days jogging. This is about two and a half years spent exercising.

How much longer would such an active person live? How many extra days of life would this diligent jogger gain in which to pursue other well-loved hobbies? We do not know for sure, but *anything* that increased average longevity by more than two and a half years in a generally healthy adult population would be considered a very large effect—a striking phenomenon. So, with two and a half years spent on the pavement, there is not likely to be much of a net gain in available time for our poor jogger. Anyone who exercised even more would gain even less, winding up with a net loss of time.

But it gets even worse. Note that in this contrived example, the unhappy jogger is trading away thousands of hours of youth for perhaps a few extra years in old age. Many individuals would not choose that trade-off. They would prefer to have their leisure time when they are young and healthy. As Neil Armstrong put it, "I believe that the Good Lord gave us a finite number of heartbeats and I'm damned if I'm going to use up mine running up and down a street."[47] Armstrong did not mind the rigorous astronaut training, but there was no way anyone was going to make him go on endless jogs.

Of course the real picture is somewhat more complicated. The jogger might really enjoy jogging and so might consider the time well spent. Or the jogger might be warding off a diagnosed tendency toward a debilitating chronic disease such as diabetes. Still, for many reasonably healthy and active individuals who are out running every morning because some advice list or some friend is pressuring them to try to improve their health, the results are not necessarily going to be what they expect. Some might have better uses for all that time, and others will be harmed by running injuries or even sudden death from cardiac arrest. This is probably why Ancel Keys spent many years doing the active gardening that he so enjoyed.

The Terman participants didn't know about running shoes, treadmills, or marathons. Few people did regular jogging or serious running before the 1960s. The Nike company didn't even exist in 1960. The Boston Marathon, the world's oldest ongoing annual marathon, had fewer than three hundred runners until 1964 (when the average Terman subject was fifty-four years old). Women could not enter the Boston Marathon until 1972 (a time when the average Terman subject was in or approaching retirement). Nowadays the Boston Marathon is usually limited to about twenty thousand runners.

From a public health point of view, it's great that so many people these days like to engage in socially hyped challenges like marathons. But it is important to recognize that these are recent social phenomena, and that many Terman participants remained steadily active in a healthy way having never even heard of a jogging trail or a spinning class.

SELF-ASSESSMENT: PHYSICAL ACTIVITY

People can be surprisingly inaccurate when asked to report how physically active they are—most tend to be positively biased, meaning that they believe they are more active than they really are. (People also tend to underestimate the number of calories they consume per day and report being a little taller and a little lighter than they actually are.) But a checklist works as a fairly realistic activity tracker.

Being as thoughtful and honest as you can, first circle each activity that you have done in the last week. Then, as accurately as you can, write the number of hours (in the last week) you spent doing the circled activities, in the blank space provided next to each.

Jogging (10-minute mile) _____	Walking moderately (3–4 mph) _____	Vacuuming _____
Swimming moderately _____	Mowing the lawn _____	Doubles tennis _____
Bicycling moderately _____	Swimming slowly _____	Moderate hiking _____
Bicycling leisurely _____	Working at the computer _____	Dog walking _____
Walking slowly (2 mph) _____	Playing a musical instrument _____	Sitting _____

Here's how to assign some approximate MET values to these activities, on a per hour basis. Jogging a 10-minute mile = 10; swimming moderately = 7; bicycling moderately = 5.5; bicycling leisurely = 3.5; walking slowly = 2.5; walking moderately = 4; mowing the lawn = 4.5; swimming slowly = 4.5; working at the computer = 2; playing a musical instrument = 2.5; vacuuming = 3.5; playing doubles tennis = 4.5; moderate hiking = 8; dog walking = 3; sitting = 1.

There are certainly activities that you have done in the past week that are not on this list. You can use the MET assignments we have listed here to estimate how many METs your other activities are worth. Assign those numbers accordingly, in an analogous fashion. Don't add in those single METs for the times when you're sleeping. Once you have done that, use the METs per hour and the total amount of time you did various activities to calculate your total METs for each activity. For example, if you walked moderately for thirty minutes every day you would have written 3.5 hours per week. Walking moderately fast is 4 METs per hour, so this would give you a total of 14 METs per week just for this one activity. Add up all the activities' totals for the week.

These METs are not tailored to an individual's level of fitness. Although walking at a pace of 3 to 4 miles per hour requires much more effort for an eighty-five-year-old grandma than it does for an eighteen-year-old member of a competitive water polo team, both the water polo competitor and the grandma will receive 4 METs. Thus, someone who is very fit will tend to overestimate his or her energy expenditure and someone who is very unfit will tend to underestimate when using this sort of a general calculation. Nonetheless, it is a useful way to quantify your approximate level of physical activity, and it is much more accurate than simply thinking, "Hmm . . . how active am I? I think I'm pretty active."

Obviously different groups of people will expend different levels of energy and so samples can be expected to vary quite a bit depending on who is included. So how do you evaluate your activity level? In one large stratified sample (meaning, chosen to be representative of the larger population) of more than fifteen thousand Europeans, the highest 20 percent expended about 250 METs or more per week while the lowest 20 percent expended less than 122 METs.[48]

Marathonlessness Is Not a Disease

If a person feels good and is a productive worker but dislikes sports and active outdoor hobbies, is that person unhealthy? One of the problems with society's overemphasis on medical diagnosis and treatment is an overclassification of illness—that is, calling too many people "sick." This peculiar problem usually arises by way of a large study finding that, on average, risk of disease or premature mortality falls with increasing exercise, lower weight, or lower blood pressure. Then some medical board sets some cutoff for abnormality—supposedly the first sign of disease. For example, a body mass index (a ratio of weight to height) that is over 30 would label you as obese.

If the "treatment" for this condition involves medication, then pharmaceutical companies chime in with strong support for a new standard. For example, it is very generally true that the higher your blood pressure, the greater your risk of heart disease and stroke. In response, the standards for normal blood pressure have been continuously lowered, with some medical boards now flatly proclaiming that normal blood pressure is "below 120/80."

Physicians used to worry when a patient's systolic blood pressure (the first number) was over 160; then the target was lowered to 150; and then for many years it was 140. Now some physicians will try adding medications to bring your blood pressure below 130 or even below 120. After all, anything higher can be called a disease, like "prehypertension." There is no doubt that bringing down very high blood pressure has saved many lives—it is one of the triumphs of modern medicine. But can things go too far? Has an illness been invented?

Something odd is going on here, because applying such ideal standards to the whole population means that the overwhelming majority of people are "sick," or at least abnormal, because they have a systolic blood pressure over 120. How can most people be abnormal? This can happen by setting a firm and arbitrary optimal standard for the population—probably a bad idea.

If you put very large numbers of people, including those who have only slightly elevated blood pressure, on various blood pressure–lowering medications for many years, a lot of them will encounter side effects. Some of these are known, but many are not. This problem gets worse because more people are on multiple medications than ever before, and the interactions or combinations of the drugs are even less well investigated or understood. Then there are the financial costs: the money being used for this medication is not being used for some other health purpose. To top it all off, it is usually the case that the added benefit of any intervention decreases as the condition becomes more mild. In other words, lowering someone's blood pressure from 160/120 to 140/100 will have a much greater impact than lowering someone's blood pressure from 130/90 to 110/70.

The same is true for physical activity and exercise. It is not yet well understood what an optimal level of physical activity should be for an average person. And it is certainly not known how to adjust such recommendations. Just as you can be too thin and your cholesterol can be too low, likewise you can exercise too much.

In fact, a tip-of-the-tail phenomenon is often ignored in medical discussions. Many studies of exercise, if you look closely, show that too much exercise can be unhealthy. Many of those exercisers at the highest part of the distribution of activity levels—those at the very tip—do not fare well. That is, physical activity definitely is associated with better health up until some point, at which many of the most active folks begin showing rising risk of injury, disease, and even premature mortality. All of which is to say that you can be perfectly healthy without being a marathon runner, and marathonlessness is not a disease.

The Risk Factor Is Not the Disease

Lest anyone accuse us authors of being lazy couch potatoes we should mention that we both enjoy outdoor activities. In fact one of us, Leslie, loves major physical challenges and ran the Marathon des Sables, something that is unusual for women to do. The Marathon des Sables is a six-day race (on foot) across the Moroccan desert, the hottest part of Africa. Runners have to carry their own food, bedding, and clothing the whole way, over 150 miles.

Nevertheless, the *predictor* of health should not be the end in itself. That is, while physical activity is associated with good health, forever increasing your physical activity to extremes will not necessarily produce better health.

Consider homocysteine, an amino acid in the blood that is a good predictor of risk of heart disease: a higher level indicates a higher risk. Folic acid and other B vitamins lower the level of homocysteine in the blood. So does taking vitamin pills with folic acid and other B vitamins dramatically reduce your risk for heart disease? The matter has been studied and, no, it probably does not help much, if at all.[49]

Again and again, careful studies reveal that markers that seem associated with good health and long life are not the primary *causes* of good health and long life. Rather, the markers are simply that—markers or indicators. Leslie enjoys some extreme sports like running the Marathon des Sables, but for personal fulfillment as part of her active lifestyle, not as a desperate attempt to secure good health.

Aspirin, Activity, and the Heart: How to Generalize

Some of Ancel Keys's long-lasting influences involved the connections he made among cholesterol, activity, and clogged arteries. In addition to eating less saturated fat, millions of people hit the running tracks and trails every morning for better heart health. As we are seeing, this is healthier than sitting around, but probably not the optimal activity for everyone.

Millions of people take an aspirin tablet daily, in a related effort to prevent a heart attack, despite the many documented and serious side effects of aspirin treatment. For some people, especially those at high risk for coronary artery blockage and who are under close supervision by their doctors, the aspirin is probably very helpful. For many others, it is probably harmful.

The first important study showing the protective effect of aspirin on those at risk for heart attack (acute myocardial infarction) was done several decades ago.[50] The participants were 1,266 male veterans. These men were not your ordinary healthy guys. They suffered from unstable angina, chest pain due to circulation problems with the heart muscle. The men in this group who were given aspirin were less likely to have a heart attack, although many did anyway. Yet most readers of this study were willing to assume that aspirin might also be helpful to nonveterans, to women, to younger people, and even to those who were not suffering from unstable angina. After all, a human body is a human body.

Subsequent studies have confirmed aspirin's value to some people but have also demonstrated its dangers. A physician who knows the at-risk patient should help make the decision in each case. Yet most have no trouble generalizing the treatment from the ill male veterans to people who are not ill male veterans. The same considerations should apply as we talk about the implications of the physical activity findings from the Terman participants. It is important to neither understate nor overstate the extent to which we can generalize findings. Just as recommendations about aspirin or about cholesterol levels have some generality but are best tailored to the individual, so, too, pathways to long life involving physical activity and associated personality and social relations are true in general, but best modified for the individual.

The Terman participants had the ability to understand medical advice and they had places to exercise. They had routine health care, and they shared many other characteristics with bright, middle-class Americans. This means that we can focus on their activity patterns, personalities, and social relations without worrying about effects of extreme poverty, ignorance, or malnutrition. But the Terman subjects, like the male veterans given aspirin, are not directly representative of the U.S. population as a whole. So we address this issue in a number of scientific ways.

First, before using scales and measures that are decades old, we carry out comparison studies using valid contemporary measures from contemporary samples of people—using metabolic equivalents (METs) to standardize activity, and modern personality scales to validate the old scales. These new comparison efforts are time-consuming but the best way to be sure that measures derived from the Terman archives are properly created and interpreted. Relatedly, and perhaps most important, we always examine our findings in the context of findings from other studies, until we are convinced that our results make sense in terms of what is more generally known.

We also use state-of-the-art statistical tests and corrections specially developed to deal with these issues. For example, we examine whether the fact that Terman limited his study to bright individuals will have an impact on the relationships among physical activity and other characteristics measured in the study. When we apply these tests and corrections, we find little or no distortion on health matters.

Even more than everyone else, we wonder about whether the lives and activities of the Terman participants are relevant to today's world. But rather than speculating, we address these issues in all of our studies and have been constantly reassured that our findings are indeed relevant.

What It Means for You: Guideposts to Health and Long Life

A half century ago, Ancel Keys said Americans should eat less and be more active. National campaigns were launched to promote physical fitness. Today almost everyone knows that fit, active people are healthier. Yet today the average American eats much more and is much less active than the average American of fifty years ago and than the average Terman subject born one hundred years ago. Advice to spend thirty minutes, at least four times per week, expending energy at the rate of 6–8 METs is good, up-to-date medical advice, but poor practical advice.

Before you take on a New Year's or birthday resolution that you are unlikely to keep, take a close look at your own past history. Our findings show that patterns of activity tend to persist over time. Look at your trajectory and at the times when you were becoming more or less active. Taking these patterns into account can help you select activities that will fit well with your preferences and lifestyle. In turn, this will make it much more likely that you'll stick with them for the long term.

If you don't like jogging, don't jog. Instead, begin doing things that you really enjoy and can keep up. It could be a long walk at lunchtime or in the evening with your friend or spouse or dog; umpiring at the local children's ball games; tending to your garden; or bowling with buddies (but not bowling alone). You don't have to do the same thing all the time, and you definitely don't have to do something that irritates or bores you.

Some say choose activities that will benefit your body *and* your soul. Others say choose something with a steady partner, for mutual support. Still others recommend team sports so that you will be pulled in by the camaraderie of the team. We recommend any or all of these and will never say "force yourself to get out there and exercise thirty minutes a day." Instead we say follow the successes of the active, healthy Terman participants: develop those patterns, whatever they are, that get you up and out of your chair.

· CHAPTER 9 ·

To Sickness or to Health?

Love, Marriage, and Divorce

In June 1940, James reported that he was happily married. He told Dr. Terman that he was very certain that no other spouse would have been as good for him. He relished his love life; and his wife, Irene, independently reported to Dr. Terman that she, too, was highly satisfied with their marriage.

About 70 percent of the Terman participants had married by this point, but one in ten of those had divorced. Barbara was one of those who had gone through a marital breakup and was now single. A caring and good-natured soul, she had happily and fully pledged her life and heart to her high school sweetheart, Fredrick. For the first year and a half everything had seemed perfect. Barbara and Fredrick both loved their jobs (she was a social worker; he was an engineer) and they shared a passion for the arts. They had several friends and enjoyed exchanging visits. They also liked playing cards, listening to music, and visiting art exhibits together in their leisure time.

As they settled into married life, though, things began to unravel. They couldn't agree on money. They clashed when it came to whether or not they should buy their own home. Barbara felt that Fredrick's constant efforts to "improve" her had hurt their marital relationship, while Fredrick complained that Barbara was a poor housekeeper and too argumentative. Before their fourth anniversary, Fredrick and Barbara had separated, and two years later their divorce was finalized. Was Barbara now at higher mortality risk?

True or False: Get Married, Live Longer?

"Married people live longer!" This adage is one of the most common conclusions to emerge from epidemiological studies of longevity. In general it is a valid description, albeit a misleading one. If you examine large western populations and compare the life expectancy of the married to the longevity of those not married, you find that married people do live longer lives. Unfortunately, this finding is often turned into the pop advice "Get married to live longer!" repeated endlessly in newspapers and magazines around the world, particularly those aimed at women. We don't know how many have taken the advice, but surely it has influenced some individuals to see spouses as health supplements as well as life partners. As with many of the other dead-end myths we've discovered, this recommendation is far, far from the truth.

It is correct that in the event of a medical emergency, it is better to have a spouse there with you to call for emergency assistance. Not only will your partner likely jump into action if you become ill, but he or she will help you understand that assistance is needed. Many who experience heart attack symptoms delay seeking treatment for critical hours; but those in the presence of a loved one are more likely to get help immediately when their symptoms kick in.

If you need to remember to take pills on time, or to stop eating that quart of ice cream, your partner can gently remind you. A spouse can help ensure cooperation with medical regimens like blood sugar testing or daily activity. On the other hand, of course, an enabling spouse might facilitate harmful behavior by bringing home an endless supply of hot dogs and beer.

If you are hospitalized, it is helpful to have an attentive family member at your bedside, advocating on your behalf. Medical errors in hospitals are a leading cause of death and disability. A hospital is one of the most dangerous places on earth, and we have known many physicians who tremble at the thought of being a patient in their own work-place. Having an advocate or even a loving and curious companion next to your hospital bed can help medical personnel catch mistakes.

A spouse can also serve as a buffer against stress. After a bad day at work, having a loving friend on hand to relax with you is very calming. But what if your spouse nags, complains, and picks at the marital scabs as soon as you walk in the door?

The point is, there is no doubt that a spouse or life partner can do many wonderful things to promote health, but such a list is not scientific evidence supporting the prescription of marriage. In fact, seeking a spouse to promote your health may not work at all!

Methodology and Marital Madness

The first flaw in the "get married to live longer" advice becomes apparent with a close reading of the relevant scientific studies. It turns out that the studies show that it is not married *people* who live longer but rather married *men*. The bulk of the evidence in various studies does not show much, if any, advantage for married women.

But there is much more. There is a well-known scale—a measure of stress—called the Social Readjustment Rating Scale. It was developed in the 1960s, though it has been updated and refined in recent years.[51] A high score on this scale epitomizes what both professionals and the lay public commonly mean when they say, "Oh, you've been under a lot of stress lately!" There is good agreement that stressful events involve such things as being fired from a job, being arrested, or losing a friend.

Accumulate enough of these nerve-racking assaults in a short period of time and your risk of illness skyrockets. The *most* stressful event is generally thought to be the death of one's spouse or life partner, but divorce ranks a close second place. (In a previous chapter we talked about parental divorce; here we are examining the effects of one's own divorce.) Divorce can devastate relations with various family members, disrupt finances, crush self-esteem, and destroy one's sense that the world is a predictable and understandable place. It is not surprising that this serious stress has long been considered relevant to health and longevity. We thus wondered about the role of divorce in the ties between marriage and long life.

Marital History

Dr. Joan Tucker, who began as a graduate student in our lab analyzing marriage and longevity and is now a leading scholar on social relations and health, helped launch our efforts to understand marriage's links to health.[52] The issue is maddening in its complexity. If marriage were like a new drug, we could give the drug to some people, and give a placebo to a group of comparison folks (the control group). But most people would not take kindly to being randomly assigned to get married.

If marriage effects were primarily physiological, like the effects of vitamin D (the sunshine vitamin), we could conduct a study like a vitamin investigation in which we compare the health of people with different diets and supplements and sun exposures, from different climates, and with different blood levels of the vitamin. But in studying marriage, we had to face the complex reasons why individuals get and stay married—a wide variety of personal reasons, social influences, and societal expectations.

Looking at the data as of the year 1950, when the Terman participants were about forty years old, Joan pointed out that while many were now married, some had previously been divorced. Others, like James, were likewise now married but still to their first spouse—we called them "steadily married." Both groups were married but had traveled different pathways—a difference worth examining.

Other Terman participants were now divorced. They had not remarried. And there was a fourth group—individuals who had always remained single. Other researchers had not been able to study marriage versus remarriage, and divorce versus singlehood across time. This division into four groups was the conceptual breakthrough we needed! Without looking at divorce and remarriage, a researcher

might erroneously miss the fact that individuals may have very different marital histories—a fact that emerged as very important.

Are You Remarried, Steadily Married, Divorced, or Steadily Single?

The Remarried Group

We began with those people who were married as of the year 1950 but
had previously been divorced. Take Philip, for example. He and Arlene
married in 1935 and soon had a daughter. Although their marriage
was bumpy at times, they always worked things out and were generally
happy. In 1941, however, Philip was called overseas, where he remained
until the end of World War II. The couple grew apart and their marriage suffered. When Philip returned home in 1945, they tried to mend
their strained relationship but finally agreed on a divorce, which was
final in 1947. Soon thereafter Philip met and married a woman he felt
"really understood" him; they were still together and doing well in
1950.

The Steadily Married Group

These people, too, were married as of 1950, but had never been divorced.
James, for example, met Irene on a blind date, set up by mutual friends.
If it wasn't "love at first sight" there was certainly a shared interest, and
they began dating steadily and exclusively within a few weeks of that
first meeting. A recent college graduate, James was employed as public
relations officer for a large international firm; he had a good income and
was ready to begin a family. When he asked Irene to marry him, just six
months after their first date, she quickly agreed. Their engagement
wasn't long—only a few months. Irene finished out that semester at college but did not return for the following term after their January wed-
ding. Instead, she set about keeping their home. Over the next five years
they had three children, whom Irene cared for at home until they began school. In 1950, with their youngest child about to enter the teen

years, James reported satisfaction with his life and his accomplishments. He was still employed with the same company and still married to the same woman.

The Divorced Group

Barbara was one of those people who had previously married but was now divorced. Like her peers in this group, she was unmarried as of midlife in 1950. After their divorce, Fredrick had moved to another state to start over, but Barbara had remained in the town where they'd lived together. She was still in the same job as a social worker and reported that being able to help people brought her a lot of joy and happiness. In fact, most of her time was devoted to her work, although she sometimes joined friends for dinner or an evening of playing cards. She also reported that she had taken up drawing—she had always loved art but hadn't seen herself as a very creative person—but after two classes she saw that she was good, particularly with charcoal. Drawing became a fun and relaxing hobby. Although Barbara viewed her failed marriage as a disappointment, she had continued to live her life and felt she hadn't suffered any real emotional problems as a result of the divorce.

In contrast, many other divorced Terman participants took things badly and remained somewhat bitter. Donna, for example—perhaps primed by the experience of her own parents' divorce—never rebounded from her own divorce into remarriage. Her trust was shaken, she was wary of relationships, and even her friendships seemed to suffer as she focused her life around supporting and raising her children.

The Steadily Single Group

These individuals had never been married. Emma, forever mature and focused, had chosen to remain single. Nevertheless, her life was quite full. After college she had spent a year abroad, staying several months with family friends in Europe and studying for a time with a well-known artist. When she returned to the United States she entered a graduate program and, after completing her Ph.D., joined the social sciences faculty at a nearby university. There, her scholarly activities kept her busy, but in her leisure time she continued to travel. Though she had not been back to Europe since that postcollege year, she had traveled extensively throughout the western United States and had made several trips east. She reported that good relationships with friends and family brought her happiness, as did her work and travels.

While they turned out to be uniquely helpful, these four groups don't account for the divergent meanings being married, remarried, divorced, or single has for men and women. So we further examined marriage and health separately for the sexes, splitting those four groups into eight. It made a huge difference.

Which Men Lived Longest?

Who lived longer, the married men or the divorced men? This is the comparison made by most studies in this field. In accord with other studies, we found that divorced Terman men were at a much higher mortality risk. The steadily married men were very likely to live to age seventy and beyond, but the divorced men were very unlikely to reach old age—fewer than a third did so!

The more fascinating comparison, however, was between the steadily married men and the remarried men. The remarried men like Philip were less likely to live long lives. They lived longer than the divorced men, but nowhere near as long as the steadily married men. Because both groups were currently married (in 1950), the marriage itself could not be the relevant protective factor. The remarried men had a wife to help with emergencies, to be at their bedside during illness, to encourage healthy habits, and to do all the other things that the wives of the steadily married men could do. So why did the remarried men die sooner?

One key reason was that they had faced the stress of divorce. As one of the greatest social stresses, the strain of divorce harms health directly, but more important, it sets in motion a series of other harmful behaviors and patterns. Ironically, advice to "get married to live longer" may *decrease* rather increase your chances for that benefit—you cannot face the stress of divorce if you have not married. Statistically, 100 percent of all divorces start with marriage.

But there is also another reason why the remarried men died sooner than the steadily married men. It involves the characteristics of the individuals who get married and stay married. We'll return to that issue in a moment.

If our explanations of these findings are correct, then steadily single men should do quite well. That is, never having to face the stress of a poor marriage and divorce, and the patterns of unhealthy behaviors that may follow, single men should lead long, healthy lives. On the other hand, single men do not enjoy the benefits of partnership we discussed earlier—help with medical regimens, assistance in recognizing and acting appropriately in a health emergency, protection in hospitals, and so on. It follows that they should fall somewhere in between the two other groups in terms of their life expectancy.

The steadily single men like John, for example, who never married, did indeed outlive the remarried group, and they way outlived the divorced men. That said, they did not, on average, live as long as the steadily married men.

Which Women Lived Longest?

Ever unpredictable, the women in the Terman study showed fascinating and unexpected results. Like their male counterparts, steadily married women lived somewhat longer lives than those women who had divorced and then remarried. The surprise emerged for women, like Barbara, who had gotten divorced and not remarried. These women didn't fare nearly as badly as did their divorced male peers. They usually lived long lives. That is, a surprising number of the women who divorced their husbands and then stayed single did fine—on average they lived nearly as long as their steadily married counterparts.

Being divorced was much less harmful to women's health than it was to men's health. This surprising finding, which had never been given much consideration before, raised many more questions about whether poor marriages could damage women's health so much that they would be better off unmarried. One thing we now knew was that simple advice to "get married to live longer" was surely flawed and incomplete.

The steadily single women were of intermediate risk. They didn't live as long as the steadily married women, but they outlived those who married and divorced and then remarried. As we later discovered, women who could thrive in a good marriage tended to stay especially healthy, but many of the rest were better off single.

As we thought more about the Terman men and women, we were pondering the H. L. Mencken saying: "Men have a much better time of it than women. For one thing, they marry later. For another thing, they die earlier."[53] Maybe Mencken was right but for the wrong reasons.

Personality, Marriage, Divorce, and Longevity

One of the best things about having the full life histories of the Terman participants is the opportunity it gave us to take a broad perspective. We weren't confined by data on marriage, divorce, or remarriage alone—we were able to go back in time and look at the pathways leading to marriage.

The Terman children who grew up to be in the steadily married group were less likely to have faced parental divorce than those in the remarried group. That is, their history with steady marriage or divorce of their parents was relevant to their own later marital history.

Parental divorce isn't nearly enough, however, to predict the potential of one's success or failure at marriage. Personality prior to marriage was directly linked to marital success. Patricia, for example, had been a conscientious and resilient child before her happy marriage to Charles. It was not marriage in isolation that would affect Patricia's long-term health and life span, but the combination and interplay of her disposition and choices.

Heading back to the data archives, our research team went in and examined the childhood personalities of the people in the different marriage and divorce groupings. We of course knew that successful marriage is not random—some individuals just don't have the temperament required for a good marriage. Indeed, when we compared the marriage groups we discovered that those folks who later became consistently married individuals had been more conscientious as children. In other words, if you were a prudent and responsible child, then you were more likely to grow up to have a successful marriage.

Our findings and interpretations of the relevance of early personality traits to marriage satisfaction squared with other studies by researchers investigating marriage and happiness. These studies have found that married people tend to be happier than unmarried people, but this is usually because people who get married tend to be happier several years before marriage; likewise, people who get divorced tend to be less happy *before* they are married.[54] Of course the marriage itself has a big impact on overall happiness but it proves imperative to examine the qualities and previous histories of those entering into marriage.

It is hard to overemphasize just how important this broader view of marriage is. When marriage is taken out of the context of the person's life pathway and viewed as an independent event, then marriage's role in health is severely distorted. For example, another study, this one of about two thousand men and women in South Carolina, likewise found divorced men were much more likely to die young than steadily married or single men. However, like us, this group of researchers found that the divorce itself was only part of the problem: there was also something about the individual characteristics and life pathways of these men that put them at risk—for both divorce and poor health.[55] We might say there are trouble-prone families.

We'd discovered that not only was marital stability relevant to long life, but that we could often predict who would have a steady marriage. The lower mortality risk of married individuals was not solely linked to the protective, helpful effects of marriage. Instead, two other dynamics entered the picture. First, marital breakup—a very stressful life event—seems tied to a long-term negative impact on health. Second, some of the so-called health advantages of being married come from influences apparent in childhood—being conscientious and not having to face the divorce of one's parents.

Recovery After a Second Marriage

You might have noticed a problem with our focus on personality and marriage success. It looks at the Terman participant but ignores his or her spouse. Yet some people divorce not because of anything about themselves but rather because they have inadvertently married trouble—someone with a personality unsuitable for a happy marriage. How could we take these issues into account?

We began by looking at the effects of divorce over a long period of time. Because many of those men who divorced later remarried, now so much the wiser, we could examine the matter again. How would such people fare in a second marriage? We looked out across the ensuing five decades at the men who remarried and then stayed married.[56] We found a tendency for the higher mortality risk of remarried men (compared with their steadily married counterparts) to decline with age. That is, the longer they lived in their remarried state, the less important the previous divorce mattered as a threat to their health.

Happiness, Marriage, and Health

It's easier to stay committed to the union if you're in a happy marriage, of course, but there are other reasons for staying hitched. Some stay married because they can't make ends meet without the spouse's second income or because they fear the financial and emotional strains of divorce itself. Others stay married for the sake of the children even though, as we saw, it is difficult to leave the children unscathed. Still others suffer in a bad relationship because they fear loneliness. The long-term effects of staying in an unhappy relationship seemed like they should have a direct correlation to health.

Were the Terman subjects in happy marriages healthier? If our explanations about marriage, stress, and health are indeed more valid than explanations simply involving help with emergencies and medications and so on, then evidence should appear in the quality of the marriages. Fortunately for us, Dr. Terman was very interested in marital and sexual satisfaction.

A half century ago, there were no good measures of marital contentment, so the ever-innovative Dr. Terman developed and validated his own new marital happiness test. He did such a good job that his scale became the basis for most modern measures of marital satisfaction.

Do you and your partner share outside interests? Do you fight about religion? Dr. Terman zeroed right in on such matters and assessed couples' preferences about spending leisure time together. He provided a list of forty activities, and the participants checked those that they really enjoyed doing and—here Terman was very clever—those that they really enjoyed doing with their spouse.

Dr. Terman also asked about regrets regarding marriage, whether the subjects had contemplated divorce, and whether they would choose the same spouse if life were to be lived over. Steadily married James checked the top of the scale; he was totally thrilled to be married to Irene. Irene was likewise delighted to be married to James, but her spousal reaction turned out to be less important to James's health.

Loryana Vie, a graduate student in our lab, helped dig deeply into these data. Working with the rest of our team, she uncovered something quite unexpected. She started by going back to the reports that James and Irene and the others had completed in 1940, astutely making use of both the Terman subjects' reports and the spouse reports.[57] Many were very happy with their marriages, many were only moderate in their satisfaction, and some were already not very happy.

Jumping forward almost a half century, we looked at the health and happiness of these people decades later. Some, like James, were very healthy, reporting good health, no cancer or heart disease, and the ability to complete daily tasks with little or no assistance. Others, in contrast, reported declining health, low energy, and serious illnesses. We also examined whether they reported a sense of well-being. Some of the participants were generally happy, satisfied with friends and with their living situation, and generally pleased with life. Others were gloomy and unhappy, listing many things they wished they had done differently in life and viewing themselves as less fortunate than their friends and colleagues.

By using our newly derived indexes, we could not only track the relations between early marital happiness and the resulting health and happiness decades later, but we could compare the effects of the husband's happiness and the wife's happiness. This is something special. Is the happiness of both partners relevant to the prediction of future health and well-being? Or perhaps it is the case, as the saying goes, that "a happy wife is a happy life"—that the wife's satisfaction is what's most important?

In general, researchers have found that the quality of one's marriage is associated with a wide range of health indicators. Not surprisingly, people in miserable marriages tend to have more symptoms and worse health.[58] But no one has looked at these effects in detail over a long period of time. To dig into these issues, Loryana focused on the marriage quality information that Dr. Terman had collected in 1940. After some searching, she discovered the original scoring keys Terman had used as well as host of relevant marriage information. We examined the wife's marital happiness, the husband's marital happiness, and the overall marital happiness of the couple. What would be the state of their health decades later?

Adding together both the husband's happiness and the wife's happiness predicted the later health of the Terman participant. But something unusual seemed to be happening when we looked over the numbers. We realized that the clearest view of the findings came when we looked not at the happiness of the couple, nor at the happiness of the individual compared to the happiness of the spouse. Instead, the key was to look exclusively at the *husband's* happiness.

The husband's marital happiness was what really mattered for later health. It was key to predicting health and well-being decades later, whether we were predicting the health of men or women. In other words, knowing that James was very happily married in 1940 let us successfully predict that James would be well decades later, but knowing that his wife, Irene, was also happily married did not add any useful information to understanding James's health. And knowing that a Terman woman's *husband* was unhappy in 1940 let us predict that she would be unhealthy and unhappy as she aged. Her own happiness when she filled out the survey in 1940 mattered much less.

Obvious simple explanations such as later divorce do not hold up. Many kinds of influences are likely coming into play. This finding does fit with other research on marriage indicating that a wife's well-being is much more affected by a difficult, hostile husband than a husband's well-being is affected by a difficult, hostile wife.[59]

Could this finding be a sign of earlier times—applicable to the Terman participants' mid-twentieth-century lives—that would no longer be true today? The question is a reasonable one, but more challenging to tackle than it first appears. Any finding that comes out of a long-term study, even a careful one, is "outdated" by the time the results come in. By definition, a forty-five-year study of married thirty-year-olds might no longer be directly relevant to the health of the next generation of thirty-year-olds. This complicated state of affairs does not mean that we can never learn anything of value. Rather, it means that we need to examine the relevant assumptions and conditions and see if they hold true in other times and places. We have already seen that many divorced women were able to thrive, and so the old stigma of divorce could not be the issue. We consider some of these matters of male-female differences later in this book.

Looking over various statistical analyses, our finding holds up quite well—a happy husband is good for the health and well-being of both the husband and the wife. As a new twist on the common wisdom that "a happy wife is a happy life," we propose: "a happy man means a healthy clan."

SELF-ASSESSMENT: MARITAL HAPPINESS

For those who are married or in a long-term relationship, the following scale assesses how happy one is with the relationship. Read each item below and circle the number that you feel best represents your feelings.

Untrue 1 2 3 4 5 completely true

1. If I had the chance to do it all over again, I would choose my same spouse (partner).   1 2 3 4 5

2. I prefer to spend any extra or unexpected leisure time with my spouse.   1 2 3 4 5

3. My marriage is extraordinarily happy.   1 2 3 4 5

4. My spouse and I share almost all of our outside interests.   1 2 3 4 5

5. I would not want to change my spouse's personality in the slightest.   1 2 3 4 5

6. My spouse and I almost always agree on family matters (such as finances and children).   1 2 3 4 5

7. My spouse and I almost always agree on matters of religion, philosophy of life, and so on.   1 2 3 4 5

8. There are many activities I enjoy doing with my spouse (such as music, travel, recreation, and so on).   1 2 3 4 5

9. My spouse is appropriately affectionate to me.   1 2 3 4 5

10. When we are alone together, my spouse and I are almost continuously delighted with each other.   1 2 3 4 5

Scoring: Each of these statements is worded in a positive direction, so there is no need for "reverse coding." Simply sum the numbers you circled—your score will range between 10 and 50. An average score on this scale is 28. The happiest spouses (those in the upper 25 percent) have scores of 35 or above, whereas those in the bottom quartile on marital happiness score at or below 19.

Sexual Activity and Satisfaction

A wife's marital satisfaction must matter in some realms. A courageous and audacious researcher, Dr. Terman wasn't afraid to ask about sexual activity. Around 1941, while reporting their marital satisfaction, the married Terman participants also revealed their sexual satisfaction and the average length of their sexual encounters. As modern researchers would later do, Terman also asked about the women's frequency of orgasm during sex. We wondered, could it be the case that a great marriage in this realm would have significant value for women's health?

Dr. Terman made sure that his field assistants were present when this touchy questionnaire was completed, in order to prevent husband and wife from collaborating or influencing each other. Fifty years later, our graduate student Dan Seldin pulled out the relevant questions and data and examined how such matters might relate to long life.

In 1941, Patricia, Charles, and the others answered many personal questions about their sex lives. Patricia might have been prudent but she was not prudish. She was asked, "How well mated are you and your husband, from the strictly sexual point of view?" Responses could range on a five-point scale from "very badly" to "no two could be more perfectly mated sexually." The average here was 3.5, somewhat above the midpoint. Patricia's response was "extremely well-mated" (a 4 on the scale). She and the other women also reported frequency of orgasm during intercourse, on a four-point scale from "never" to "always." The average was 2.8, again revealing a generally good but not outstanding sexual satisfaction. And Patricia was again near the top.

These answers allowed us to create a predictor measuring what Dr. Terman called "orgasm adequacy of wives."[60] We looked to see if this sexual satisfaction would be related to a longer life, after taking the women's personalities into account. Women who had a higher frequency of achieving orgasm during intercourse tended to live longer than their less fulfilled peers.[61]

We—and lots of women out there—wish we knew why. The limited sexual information available from other studies does suggest an association between sexual activity and health, in both men and women, but the links are hazy.[62] There is a dearth of scientific information available on sexual fulfillment and long-term health, not really so surprising when one imagines what it must be like going to a government-funded research agency to ask for money to study orgasms and health. Here's what we do know. Sexual satisfaction tends to play a role in a happier marriage, and happier marriages play a role in greater sexual satisfaction (a chicken-and-egg dilemma). And we know that people in stable, fulfilling marriages tend to be healthier. What is causing what? We won't know until the completion of other long-term studies of intimacy, personality, behavior, and health. At the moment, we can say that a sexually satisfying and happy marriage is a very good indicator of future health and long life.

What It Means for You: Guideposts to Health and Long Life

To sickness or to health? What can we make of all these findings about marriage, divorce, remarriage, and health and long life? First, if you are a single woman with a number of friends and an interesting life, don't think you need to follow the misleading suggestion to get married (or remarried) to improve your health. Women, like Barbara, who had gotten divorced and not remarried usually lived long lives—on average they lived nearly as long as their steadily married counterparts. And contrary to all the popular advice, our research shows that being single can often be just as healthy for a woman as being in a marriage—particularly if she has been stably, consistently single and has other fulfilling social relationships such as close friendships, meaningful memberships in organizations, and family ties.

Married men do live longer but usually only if they are suited to a lasting marriage and do not divorce. Those who were prudent and responsible as children and those from stable homes were more likely to grow up to have a successful marriage. So here, too, seeing marriage as an element you need for long life is a gross oversimplification—it depends an awful lot on the particular man and the marriage.

Those well-adjusted people who have found a long-term compatible partner are likely to live significantly longer than their peers who are only sometimes attached, particularly if they are men. Those who find their relationships repeatedly dissolving, even into their forties and fifties, could face significant health risks. If that describes you, pay special attention to the information about careers and social organizations in the following chapters.

Happiness in couples is generally a sign of good health to come, but it is the man's happiness that most especially predicts the couple's later health. This was true for the Terman participants and the finding is being confirmed by modern physiological research.

We also wanted to look at the later effects of being widowed—was this more of a problem for the women or the men? We take up this matter in our analysis of masculinity, femininity, and long life. But first we needed to understand more about healthy careers.

CHAPTER 10

Careers, Success, and Satisfaction

Thriving and Surviving

E dward Dmytryk, the highly successful director of *The Caine Mutiny* (starring Humphrey Bogart, in 1954), had anything but an easy, unstressful life. He was the son of Ukrainian immigrants who had moved the family to San Francisco (and then Los Angeles) just in time for the young Edward to be noticed by his teacher and recommended to Terman for the newly launching study. A few years later, Edward left home as a teenager and struck out on his own to work as a low-paid messenger at Paramount Pictures. As he worked his way up in the film industry, Edward continued to face many remarkable challenges.

Mr. Dmytryk's movie career stopped abruptly in 1947 when he was called before the House Un-American Activities Committee, which was investigating Communists and Communist sympathizers in Hollywood. Defending his freedom of thought and action, Dmytryk refused to testify and became one of the "Hollywood 10"—the directors and producers who were cited for contempt of Congress.[63] He was sent to a federal prison camp, and his wife divorced him the following year.

In 1951 Dmytryk, who had been blacklisted and was unable to work in Hollywood, decided to change his stance and testify after all. He went back to the committee and confirmed that he and a number of other silent witnesses had indeed been previously involved with the Communist Party. For many years later, some in Hollywood scorned him as a sellout and informer. Others disdained him as a former Communist. Yet his career was spectacularly successful. In addition to *The Caine Mutiny*, he went on to direct such stars as Spencer Tracy, Deborah Kerr, Clark Gable, Elizabeth Taylor, Marlon Brando, and Richard Burton. One of the publicly identified of Dr. Terman's subjects, Dmytryk lived almost the full twentieth century, dying at age ninety on July 1, 1999. How could someone facing such a stressful life and career live a long and healthy life?

Stress Is Not All It's Cracked Up to Be

"Relax," "avoid stress," "don't work too hard"—these are common exhortations for staying healthy—but turn out to be poor advice. Another dead-end myth. There is no evidence that people told to relax necessarily become healthier as a result. (We are not talking here of course about someone who is seriously ill and needs bed rest.) Could it be that if you give up an interesting, demanding job to retire and move away from your friends to live in a warm-weather golf community you may be *increasing* the risk to your health?

When scientists throw rats together in an overcrowded, competitive cage, the rats get sick. A problem with referring to the stresses of modern life as a "rat race" is that it makes us too willing to believe that what is bad for rats is bad for people. Interestingly, we rarely think the opposite—that what is good for rats is good for people. Few of us envy the life of a happy rat. The fundamentals of learning—rewards and punishments—are similar in rats and humans, but there are vast differences in overall brain function and social interactions.

In humans, there is little or no direct substantiation that the challenges of daily life on the job suppress the immune system and thereby cause significant numbers of people to die from cancer and other immune-related diseases.[64] Similarly, there is little or no evidence that people who are heavily involved in their jobs or work long hours are more prone to heart disease. It all depends on what kinds of stresses you face and on how you deal with them.

This does not mean that unbearable stress over long periods of time is not a problem. People such as combat veterans who have encountered more horror than they can cope with may very likely face post-traumatic stress disorder (PTSD). Those with PTSD suffer significant sleep disruptions (such as nightmares), chronic irritability, and problems expressing feelings, which lead to both internal disruptions and problems with families and other social relations. As we will see in chapter 14, in which we examine the Terman men who went to war, PTSD sufferers may also develop related unhealthy patterns—drinking heavily or abusing prescription or illegal drugs.

Some people face similar significant stress after years of workplace harassment. Clearly these things lead to significant health problems. But it is important to distinguish between severe, chronic stress reactions and the usual kinds of "stress" we find at work or school.

Healthy Careers?

In 1940, when the popular and cheerful Paul was thirty-three years old, he reported his career triumphs and challenges to Dr. Terman. And he'd already had plenty of both. In college Paul had been active in journalism, working on the campus newspaper and writing short stories for a literary society. A real extrovert, he loved interviewing people and digging into their histories. Always the optimist, Paul had taken a low-level position at a local newspaper following graduation. He knew he wouldn't have the best assignments right off, but he felt certain he would work his way to the top.

The job wasn't all Paul had hoped it would be, though. He wanted to write human interest stories and found himself frustrated with constant pieces on product comparisons and economic trends. He stuck it out for nearly three years before resigning. Over the next several years he held various positions (salesman, proofreader, typist) and finally found himself, in 1940, as the manager of a large bookstore. He reported to Dr. Terman that, although he had "drifted into" his current line of work, he liked it very much; he envisioned new ways of

connecting the bookstore to the larger community, such as by bringing well-known authors to do readings and book signings and by high-
lighting local writers. But when asked, "Have you definitely chosen
your life work?" Paul couldn't say with any certainty.

In contrast, John, the active and shy scientist, was quite certain
he'd picked the right vocation. At the time of the 1940 assessment,
John had been out of school for only two years—he had been completing a postdoctoral fellowship in physics and had just recently taken a
faculty position at a prestigious California university. His career path
showed a high degree of dedication and perseverance, consistent with
his having been rated as very conscientious by his teacher in 1922.
John was enthusiastic about his job, stating that he had "definitely
chosen" his occupation and life work. He described his work as very
fulfilling, not only because it suited his temperament but also because
it was a way to serve society. Physicists were in great demand as the
United States geared up to compete in a world that was rapidly indus-
trializing and heading for war.

Many of the Terman participants were professionals like John—
lawyers, engineers, physicians, professors, or teachers. Many others, like
Paul, wound up in business—in banking, accounting, advertising, and
as managers of all sorts. Still others were spectacularly unsuccessful.
Some were chronically unemployed. About a quarter of the men found
work in less prestigious jobs—clerical workers, salesmen, craftsmen,
and so on. Certainly nothing to be ashamed of, but nowhere near
matching the early potential that brought them into the study. Dr. Terman, however, was singularly unimpressed. He even sniffed about a few
of these cases of low-status workers by reporting that their leisure time
was "devoted to writing of doubtful promise."[65] Perhaps they believed
they were writing the Great American Novel, but Terman was neither
pleased nor awed, seeing absolutely no evidence of a rising sun.

Because of the limited career options for the women of this time
period, we follow Terman's lead here and focus primarily on the men.
Although about half of the Terman women had jobs outside the home
at some point, most senior occupational positions were closed to
women, and so their job titles were misleading. We did, however, look

at the many individual career paths of the women, and the findings generally were in line with what we saw in the men.

Career Success

Edward, Paul, John, and all the other Terman men were very different in their career paths and successes. They diverged quite a bit in the demands and stresses their careers entailed. Yes, Edward Dmytryk, the highly successful but highly stressed Hollywood director, lived to age ninety, but many stressed others took ill and died young. Puzzled, we wanted to know if there was a general pattern, and if so, what caused it.

Two questions jumped out at us. First, did the men who worked hard, fought to overcome many obstacles, and achieved high status and demanding positions suffer health problems and early death? And did those men in the less demanding jobs find the paths to long life? Remember that all of the participants were intelligent, promising students at around age eleven, and so probably all had the potential to have a highly successful career.

Second, how did the match between one's inclinations and one's career influence later health and longevity? Would those whose jobs fit their personalities live longer? That is, would the artistic child who, yielding to the pressures of his father, became an engineer be frustrated and at an especially high health risk?

Because Terman was especially interested in the future success and leadership contributions of the bright and able children, he spent a lot of time and effort collecting information on their subsequent careers and achievements. Based on their achievements by young adulthood (mostly in their early thirties) Terman and his fellow experts evaluated whether the men had lived up to their high potential. Terman enlisted a longtime vocational counselor to assist him in making these judgments—someone with much practical knowledge of occupational fields. Rather than relying on a single, potentially misleading measure like income, Terman looked at a variety of factors. For example, if you were a businessman, then your income was certainly taken into consideration, but if you were a college professor with a brilliant record but low income, you were still categorized as successful.

Some of the classification was easy. If you were listed in *Who's Who in America*, you were put down as highly successful. If you were a prominent doctor or lawyer, you likewise made the cut for the top group. A few Terman subjects were already quite accomplished in art, film, or radio. By the mid 1940s, the Terman participants had published almost one hundred books and hundreds of articles, poems, and short stories.

In the end, about one-fifth of the men were classified as highly successful. Another one-fifth were deemed unsuccessful. The rest were somewhere in between. Not all of the unsuccessful men were in non-professional or low-status careers. Some were chemists, teachers, or engineers but not very accomplished at what they did. Others were even lower on the rungs of occupational status. One was a baker, one was a letter carrier, one was a porter, and one was a streetcar conductor. As Terman insisted, none of these men lacked the intelligence to perform a higher-status job.

Is Nuclear Physics Easy and Relaxing?

Norris Bradbury, who has been publicly identified as a Terman participant, became an atomic physicist and played a key role working on the Manhattan Project, the crash program to build the first atom bomb. He succeeded J. Robert Oppenheimer as director of Los Alamos National Laboratory, a job he was very hesitant about taking and yet kept for decades. It is hard to imagine a more high-pressure job than overseeing the development of the nation's nuclear arsenal at a time of severe Cold War tension and threats. Did it eventually enfeeble Bradbury?

Not at all. In 1970 the Atomic Energy Commission presented Mr. Bradbury its highest honor, the Enrico Fermi Award. He was tremendously successful in his long career. And, despite all the stresses and challenges, Bradbury lived a very long life—to age eighty-eight. He was survived by his wife of sixty-four years (Lois Platt Bradbury), three children, seven grandchildren, and four great-grandchildren.[66]

Although Terman was very pleased with the striking success of many, he warned that future ill health or other misfortune might disrupt the highly promising careers of even his most successful participants. What he did *not* foresee was that health threats could be predicted by career accomplishments. Or, as was more often the case, by lack of accomplishments.

Studying Success and Longevity

More than a half century after Terman collected his data on occupational success (data collected on about seven hundred men) we looked into the long-term consequences on health and longevity. Would Paul's easygoing, free-flowing approach to his career as a bookstore manager be a benefit or a curse? Would John's dedication to physics lead to a stressful but long life like that of fellow physicist Norris Bradbury, or was Bradbury's long life an anomaly—an exception to the rule?

We gathered together our collaborators and research assistants, filling our computer programs with a whole host of relevant information, including the personality indexes we had constructed and validated earlier. We recorded how much alcohol the men drank, the participants' reports of their ambition, and even their parents' reports of how driven they thought their sons to be. Most important, we used the death certificates to see how long they lived.

The Press to Success Doesn't Kill You, It Makes You Stronger

The results were very clear: those with the most career success were the least likely to die young. In fact, on average the most successful men lived five years longer than the least successful![67]

The Terman subjects who were moderately successful lived longer than the less successful, but not as long as the more successful. Epidemiologists call this a dose-response relationship—the greater the dose of success, the longer the life.

Especially convincing about this finding is that the men who were independently rated by Terman as most successful more than a half century ago were the ones least likely to die at any given age in the decades that followed. Some studies in this field of research might be inadvertently biased by the classifications or judgments used by the epidemiologists, but in this case, we did not have to do any job classifications or make any judgments—we simply relied on those careful categorizations Terman and his associates had made decades ago.

Why the Successful Live Longer

Everyone knows that the rich tend to live longer than the poor, and we often think that we know why. People think that access to the best doctors, the fanciest gyms, and the safest homes make the difference. In some cases this is certainly very true. Those mired in poverty face a whole host of significant health threats. But much more is going on below the surface.

One matter that continues to stump researchers, for example, is why those in the upper middle class tend to live longer than those in the middle class, when both have enough food, housing, and medical care. Our study of the Terman participants examined this question in a very different way from the standard rich-versus-poor or favored-versus-deprived approach. In our study, we had a mostly advantaged, middle-class, educated sample of people, and yet the highly successful long outlived their very bright peers who were less successful. If their surroundings were alike, then, we wondered, could it perhaps be their individual personalities that accounted for the difference?

Conscientiousness, as we have established, is a strong predictor of longevity, and it turns out that the professionally successful Terman subjects were indeed more conscientious than their peers. But conscientiousness didn't explain everything: those with a successful career lived much longer even after taking their conscientiousness into account.

Conscientiousness did, however, make a big difference for those who were least successful in their careers. Those men who were very unsuccessful in their careers and who were also very unconscientious (on their childhood assessments) had a whopping increase in their mortality risk. If you were both unconscientious and unsuccessful, you were especially likely to die before reaching even age sixty.

Not surprisingly, ambition predicted career success. More to the point, ambition, coupled with perseverance, impulse control, and high motivation, was not only good for achievement but was part of the package of a resilient work life. It is not a coincidence that Edward Dmytryk was a prominent director and lived a long life or that Norris Bradbury headed a powerful agency and lived a long life. Symphony conductors, company presidents, and bosses of all sorts tend to live longer than their subordinates.

Complementing our own analyses, the sociologist Glen Elder and his colleagues looked at career changes between 1940 and 1960 and found evidence that the Terman men who moved among various jobs without a clear progression were less likely to live long lives than those with steadily increasing responsibilities in their field.[68] In other words, a stable and successful career is often part and parcel of a successful pathway to long life. Usually this increasing responsibility brings more challenges and a heavier workload, but paradoxically this is *helpful* to long-term health.

The Real Source of Workplace Stress

Converging evidence from a number of studies suggest that the damaging sort of workplace stress arises from conflicts with other people rather than from the challenges and demands of the work itself. Having a poor relationship with your overbearing boss can lead to health problems, and not getting along with your coworkers can be quite harmful. This is especially true if you have lots of responsibilities that depend on the cooperation of others but you do not have the resources or the leadership qualities to make things happen. On the other hand, if you have resources and a good deal of influence over outcomes, demanding tasks will be less stressful for you. It makes sense that those agency heads, symphony conductors, and company presidents who have both power and leadership skills will tend to remain healthy despite very demanding careers.

Individuals who tend to react with hostility to interpersonal slights are particularly likely to suffer lingering physiological damage. Those Terman subjects who were less critical of others, tried to avoid arguments, and didn't always try to get things their own way tended to be healthier and live longer. John, Norris, and others did not shy away from controversy but did seek out the good in other people. In fact, Edward Dmytryk blamed his good intentions and his desire for solidarity with the others of the Hollywood 10 for his early affiliation with the Communist Party, which he was later quick to abandon.

To some extent unhealthy behaviors and circumstances—more smoking and drinking, and less stable marriages—played a role in the unsuccessful Terman subjects' earlier deaths, but the core problem of being unconscientious and unsuccessful remained even for those who never chose partying over work. It was something deeper about how they lived their lives that led them to die sooner. Unsuccessful Terman subjects who had been characterized as having comparatively low motivation even in childhood were at greater mortality risk than successful individuals.

In the early 1970s—a half century into the study—the Terman men who were still alive were in their sixties, and their working lives, including occupational achievement and work satisfaction, were again assessed in some detail.[69] The first thing that was clear was that work and family were the most important aspects of life for the Terman men, more so than friends or the pursuit of culture or happiness. Work was not seen as stress to be shunned but was highly valued.

But what predicted their degree of work satisfaction? Those, like John, who had earlier (in 1940) felt that they had chosen their occupation (rather than drifted into it) were much more satisfied. Further, those who had always been more ambitious and liked the challenges of work were more satisfied as they approached their retirement years.

What About the Women?

Melita Mary Hogg Oden was born in 1898 in Saratoga, California, and attended college twenty miles up the road at Stanford University. Fortunately for Melita, Stanford, which was a new school in fast-growing California, happened to be one of the few private colleges to admit both men and women. She studied psychology and graduated in 1921, just as Lewis Terman was launching his major project. Melita was recruited to assist, and she spent the next four decades at Terman's side.[70]

In Dr. Terman's first published works, Melita is not mentioned, although by his 1930 book *The Promise of Youth*, she is credited as an assistant. But by the time of the major 1947 book *The Gifted Child Grows Up: Twenty-five Years' Follow-up of a Superior Group*, Melita Oden is the coauthor. Still, even in this volume, Terman writes in the preface, "Mrs. Oden has served continuously as my research associate in the follow-up study of the group since 1936,"[71] and goes on to thank her for checking "the typed characters against manuscript copy" and for reading the printer's proof.

Some hint of the major—and understated—contributions of Melita Oden to the Terman project comes from her activities after Lewis Terman died, when she returned to Saratoga. There she helped found the Saratoga Historical Foundation and became its historian, a position she held for many years. She kept extensive and meticulous records about Saratoga until her death in 1993. Widowed in 1959, she thrived for decades and was named Saratoga "Citizen of the Year" for 1976. In today's world, of course, Melita Oden would have become a professor herself, not merely Terman's essential and eternal research assistant.

Melita was not a Terman subject, but her life history parallels those of a lot of the female Terman participants. Many were highly successful, but within the limits that society imposed on them. Because their career titles were often misleading or meaningless, we could not formally examine the careers and longevity of the women. But our sense is that the results would have been analogous to those of the men. Melita Oden—bright, hardworking, well educated, very meticulous, and highly accomplished—lived in good health until she died at age ninety-five.

Shelley Smith Mydans is an outstanding example of how career success and longevity go together. Shelley, the *Life* magazine reporter we met at the beginning of the book, was captured by the Japanese in Manila while covering World War II. Her career in journalism was always challenging but very successful. Assigned first to Europe in 1939 and then to cover the Sino-Japanese War and then to Manila, she spent two years in captivity until her release in a prisoner exchange. One of Shelley's duties while in prison camp was to pick the weevils out of the cereal.[72]

She later returned to overseas correspondence, working in radio news and reporting for *Time*. In her spare time, she wrote (and published) novels. Shelley Smith Mydans had a very challenging but highly successful career, as well as a successful marriage and children. It is said that she faced more stressful adventures than a soldier of fortune. Yet she lived a long, healthy life, dying in 2002 at age eighty-six.

SELF-ASSESSMENT: JOB PASSION AND ACCOMPLISHMENT

For each of the statements in the left-hand column, circle the description on the right that most accurately reflects your feeling.

1. When I work, my productivity is high.

   1 – This is occasionally true of me
   2 – This is sometimes true of me
   3 – This is often true of me
   4 – This is almost always true of me

2. I feel that my work is meaningful.

1 – Almost always
2 – Often
3 – Sometimes
4 – Occasionally

3. An important goal of my life is to reach the point where I can stop working and relax for a change.

1 – It is a minor goal
2 – It is a moderately important goal
3 – It is a very important goal
4 – It is the most important goal

4. My career success depends on my efforts, not on luck.

1 – I feel this way once in a while
2 – I feel this way about half the time
3 – I often feel this way
4 – I almost always feel this way

5. There is a lot I still want to accomplish in my career.

1 – Absolutely; I still have many career-related goals
2 – There are some things I still want to do
3 – There are only a few things I still want to do
4 – I've accomplished enough in my career and now I can relax

6. In the past decade, I have received special honors or awards.

1 – Yes, I often receive such recognition
2 – Yes, my efforts and contributions are sometimes specially recognized
3 – No, I am usually not that willing or able to be singled out for achievement
4 – No, I am never singled out for special accomplishments

7. In whatever I do, I aspire to excellence much more than do my colleagues.

1 – Not really
2 – Sometimes
3 – Most of the time
4 – Definitely

8. Promotions are at the whim of my boss and not really under my control.

1 – Definitely true
2 – Probably true
3 – Maybe true
4 – Not at all true

9. I am passionate about the job that I do.

1 – Not really
2 – Partly
3 – Mostly
4 – Without a doubt

To score this scale, first reverse the numerical value for statements 2, 3, 5, and 6. So, on number 2, if you said "almost always," a 1, change it to a 4. Similarly, for these four questions change 2s to 3s, change 3s to 2s, and change 4s to 1s. Once you have done that, simply sum the values. Your score should fall somewhere between 9 and 36, with higher numbers reflecting a greater sense of passion, accomplishment, and control in one's occupation. About 25 percent of people are expected to score above 25, while the lowest 25 percent will score around 16 and below. High scorers, despite sometimes feeling overwhelmed by the demands of their job, sense the rewards of their work and may see additional payoff in terms of longer lives.

Mismatching

We regularly chat with college students and young professionals who are searching for their ideal career paths. They are looking for a "match" between their own characteristics and the demands of their eventual careers, believing that if they fail to choose the right occupation they will be unhappy and unhealthy.

We have developed a concept that applies to this situation—the notion of a "self-healing personality." This is the idea that a good match between an individual's personality and the demands of one's environment is a path to mental and physical health. For example, there is no sense in forcing an athletic student who loves roughhousing, an intelligent student who loves reading books, and an extroverted student who loves leadership all to pursue the same after-school activities. It would be better for them to choose according to their abilities and interests. We predicted that Terman men whose personalities fit well with their jobs would live longer. It made great intuitive sense to us, but was it true? It turned out to be more complicated.

Over the course of a career, the average worker spends tens of thousands of hours dedicated to his or her occupation. Psychologist John Holland created one of the most well-tested and widely used systems for simultaneously categorizing individuals according to both personality type and occupational environment.[73] Holland believed that the choice of a vocation is often an expression of personality and so developed a framework that was ideal for seeing what happens when people work (or do not work) in fields that fit them.

Holland defined six types that refer both to individuals and to occupations. *Artistic* people and artistic occupations include actors, musicians, designers, and artists. *Realistic* occupations are those where people "do" things—engineers, firefighters, pilots, machinists, veterinarians, and so on. *Investigative* occupations involve a lot of thinking—economists, professors, and chemists. *Social* occupations include helpers such as clergy, nurses, teachers, and counselors. *Enterprising* careers generally involve persuasion such as insurance, politics, and general sales. *Conventional* occupations emphasize organizational skills, such as administration, financial analysis, and auditing. There is some overlap among these categories but they do a good job of capturing the general emphases of occupational skills, tasks, and interests.

Applying Holland's categories to the Terman archives, our team (initially motivated by then–graduate student Kathleen Clark) gathered and coded information from 1940 about each person's likes, dislikes, occupational interest scores, and preferences for various pursuits.

We analyzed about four hundred activities, looking for whether the Terman men worked in occupations that matched their own personality characteristics or whether they had, for various reasons, not worked in their compatible fields.

We predicted that those individuals who spent their lives working in occupations that were a good fit for their interests would face less stress and so would be healthier and live longer. We expected that individuals who loved and valued artistic activities would be healthiest if they worked in an artistic field and least healthy if they became, say, financial analysts.

In fact, however, being well suited to one's job did not always predict a longer life. A match could actually be a health risk factor. Among men in the Enterprising group, those with high congruence between personality and occupation died sooner—assertive, persuasive men who worked in occupations such as sales management were at greater risk than assertive, persuasive men working in other types of occupations. The personality predisposition and the career reinforced each other, bringing out the stresses and unhealthy habits common to each.

Men who were less enterprising (in terms of their personalities) but found themselves holding enterprising jobs were also at relatively high mortality risk. The stressful enterprising jobs brought out latent unhealthy tendencies and they faced more stress and poorer health habits. But the less enterprising still weren't as badly off as the "always on" personalities working in jobs that required them to be go-getters.

The one case in which a good career-to-personality match was helpful was the Social category. Men with social personality types (co-operative and having good people skills) who were working in social environments (like counseling) did live longer.

Overall, our findings revealed that when choosing a career, finding the "perfect match" doesn't necessarily put one on a path toward long life. This doesn't mean that choosing one's career path is unimportant. All of us have things that we detest doing, and naturally it would not be smart to intentionally choose a job that requires these activities day after day, year after year. But living out one's dreams was not what led to health and longevity. It was a productive perseverance, a sense of mastery and accomplishment buoyed by one's career successes, that did that. We hope this is a comforting finding for students and young people on the brink of life-shaping career choices.

Aging, Productivity, and Health

But what about older participants? What were the impacts of productivity on long life for those who had already completed the most rigorous part of their career? We looked to the 720 Terman participants—both men and women—who were still alive in the 1980s, at which time most were over seventy years old. We studied whether each person was still productive, motivated, and accomplishing things. Some of the Terman participants continued to work for pay, either part-time or full-time. Others were pursuing new educational opportunities or setting new goals and achieving new awards. Some were motivated to work for social change or make a new contribution to society. We compared those who were highly productive in old age to those who were taking it easy and were not so concerned with racking up accomplishments.

The findings were dramatic. Looking over the next two decades, the continually productive men and women lived much longer than their more laid-back comrades. This productive orientation mattered more than their social relationships or their sense of happiness and well-being.[74]

Again, it was their prudence, dependability, and perseverance that made the difference. The highly productive elderly Terman subjects were those who, earlier in life, had been assessed as the most conscientious. They were also less likely to be heavy drinkers or carousers. It was not the happiest or the most relaxed older participants who lived the longest. It was those who were most engaged in pursuing their goals.

But Were They Happy?

Skeptics might wonder whether hard workers are really enjoying life. Are they missing out on enjoying the good things? Just as we previously found that conscientious, dependable people are not leading boring and stale lives, we now found that productive, hardworking people (even in old age) are not stressed and miserable, but tend to be happier, healthier, and more socially connected than their less productive peers.

Other researchers have found the same thing (though not via life-span studies): People who have meaningful and important jobs and who are especially productive are much happier than those who are unpressured, lackadaisical slackers.[75] People on the right pathways to long life work harder in their jobs. And they not only stay healthier but they are happier to boot. People like Norris Bradbury, Edward Dmytryk, and Shelley Smith Mydans are thrivers and survivors.

Is Education the Key?

In the classic film *The Wizard of Oz*, the Scarecrow complains resentfully that he has only straw in his head but no brains. Yet as he and the other characters journey down the Yellow Brick Road to seek help from the Wizard, the Scarecrow repeatedly behaves in a clever and wise manner, with many excellent ideas.

When the characters finally reach the Land of Oz, the Wizard says to the Scarecrow, "Anybody can have a brain." The Wizard even helpfully points out that universities are full of professors who think deep thoughts "with no more brains than you have." But the Wizard then admits to the Scarecrow that wise, successful, and well-educated individuals "have one thing you haven't got—a diploma!" So he presents a diploma and the *expectations* that go along with it. With the proper credentials in hand, a bright individual not only has the capacity to succeed but has the motivation and confidence to thrive.

The better-educated Terman participants did tend to live longer than their equally bright peers. But as we described in chapter 6, level of education was not a strong predictor of later health and longevity, especially as compared to other individual, social, and career predictors. Rather, it was the high expectations, perseverance, and the patterns of accomplishment that were important.

If you are better educated and more productive in life—successful at work and likely to continue to grow and be creative—the success flows over into other domains of your life. This means that education per se is not enough. Instead, it is becoming the kind of person who is able and motivated to take the helm through life's personal and social passages that makes the biggest difference.

What It Means for You: Guideposts to Health and Long Life

Edward Dmytryk's mother died when he was very young, and he had a rough childhood. He lived a life full of great challenges and great successes and now rests in Forest Lawn Cemetery in the Hollywood Hills of Los Angeles. He lived ninety years and his films will live on for many more. Mr. Dmytryk and his fellow hardworking, stressed, but successful Terman subjects were the ones who thrived. It was not at all the case that hard work was unhealthy, and it was not at all true that the long-lived led uninteresting lives.

Like Shelley Smith Mydans, many of the long-living Terman participants faced times when they had to do such things as pick weevils out of their cereal. What our research makes clear is that working hard to overcome adversity or biting off more than you can chew—and then chewing it—does not generally pose a health risk. Striving to accomplish your goals, setting new aims when milestones are reached, and staying engaged and productive are exactly what those following the guideposts to a long life tend to do. The long-lived didn't shy away from hard work for fear that the stress of it would lead to an early demise; the exact opposite seems true!

Finding the perfect career to match your personality and preferences is not the way to guarantee success or long life. Many Terman subjects found themselves in less-than-ideal jobs and yet attained great success and satisfaction. Others who did find a perfect career match ended up risking their health because occupational demands accentuated their natural tendencies toward unhealthy patterns. Instead of their smarts or the career counseling they received, it was their spirited drive and take-charge attitude that spurred the successful Terman participants toward accomplishment and, surprisingly, to especially long lives.

What the Wizard said to the Scarecrow, "Anybody can have a brain," could just as easily have been something Dr. Terman said to his subjects. They were all quite smart, but this was not enough to take them very far. Being intelligent was not a ticket to long life, but channeling knowledge and smarts toward productive achievement was.

· CHAPTER 11 ·

Long Life Meets the Afterlife

Religion and Health

Religion played a different role in Linda's, John's, and Donna's lives. Linda was raised Catholic and attended Sunday school most weeks. At age twenty, she married a Catholic man and they remained active together in their church throughout their lives. John, in contrast, lived pretty much without religious involvement. As a young adult, he focused on his career and never developed an interest in congregational religion. Donna was more representative of most of the Terman participants: in her twenties she was somewhat interested in her Lutheran church, and during the decade that followed she became further involved, bringing her children to Sunday school. She was never as devoted as Linda, however, and her religious involvement gradually waned as her children grew up and left home.

Was religious involvement relevant to the health and long life of the Terman participants? Overall in the United States, we know that religious people tend to be healthier and live somewhat longer than the nonreligious, but there is a lot of individual variation.[76] Similar results have emerged from other studies in Europe and Asia. Why do religious folks stay healthier and live longer? Does praying make a difference?

Ancient advice about long life comes from the biblical book of Exodus, where one of the Ten Commandments instructs, "Honor your father and your mother so that you may have a long life in the land which the Lord God is giving you." Among the many commentaries on this stark verse, three are highly relevant to the issue of religion and health. The first interpretation is that those who live a righteous life will be blessed with long life. A second, alternative interpretation asserts that the honoring of parents is necessary for the nation (or people) to remain in the Holy Land. A third interpretation is that a harmonious, respectful family life and social structure will lead to a stable civilization and long healthy lives. These age-old thoughts turned out to provide an excellent framework for our modern thinking about families, religion, social relations, and health.

Sometimes religion can be dangerous to health. People who shun modern medical treatment in favor of faith healing can cause great harm to themselves or their ill family members. A few religious groups have become cults that advocate violence or antiscientific practices. But such groups are a minority, and we are focusing our research attention on mainstream religious organizations that are compatible with modern life and scientific knowledge.

Does Prayer Work?

People often ask us if praying leads to better health and longer life. The questioner may be asking either if religious devotion and the associated psychosocial characteristics affect health or if intercessory prayer does. There have been a number of studies on intercessory prayer—examining whether praying for a sick person can lead to recovery via divine intervention. Some of them try to be very scientific. That is, they may have a control group (a comparison group) of ill people who are not prayed for. But it would be disappointing for many ill folks to know that no one is praying for them. So a study may go even further and be a double-blind study, in which neither the doctor nor the patient knows who is being systematically prayed for and who is not. Intellectual interest in such matters traces back several hundred years to the Scottish philosopher David Hume, who wrote about the reasoning and evidence needed to establish the existence of miracles.[77]

From a psychological point of view, these arguments are fascinating. Most proponents of intercessory prayer present it as an article of faith. For most scientists, however, faith in supernatural forces is outside their realm. This does not mean that scientists cannot have faith in the supernatural, just that such ideas depend wholly upon, well, faith. By definition, *supernatural* means "beyond the natural," and unexplainable by scientific law.

So why would someone design a scientific experiment to try to test an article of faith? We think that such attempts arise repeatedly in a society that is too willing to underestimate the psychological, social, and behavioral influences on health and well-being. Because the "science" of modern medicine is often too quick to reduce health to simple mechanical cause-and-effect relations, many patients feel a dissatisfaction and frustration with medical care. They "know" that a good family life (honoring father and mother) and devotion to others can lead to good health. Our studies of the Terman participants, as well as studies by others, convinced us that good health is indeed a much more complicated phenomenon and that religion provides a good insight into pathways to long life.

Religious Involvement Throughout Life

In 1950 Donna and the other Terman participants (who were then around forty years old) were asked, "As an adult, to what extent are you religiously inclined?" Some were not at all religiously inclined, others were a little, and still others were moderately or strongly religious. Donna, for example, indicated that she was moderately religious. The question did not ask respondents if they were affiliated with a particular religion or regularly attended religious services. Instead this was a more global question, accounting for private practice of religion, too.

Unfortunately, a particular type of bias often crops up in studies of religion and health: people who report that they attend religious services on a regular basis may be healthier to start with—they have the ability to get out and about, they are not severely depressed, and they have enough social skills to be able to function in a community. We designed our studies to look at health effects that go beyond these obvious ones.

The cases of Linda and John and Donna showed us that religious involvement has many aspects that could be relevant to good health, but they also illustrated the differences among individuals in their religious devotion and their daily health habits. Linda was both the most traditional and the most religious of the three. She had a compassionate nature, being described in childhood as "kind on principle" and unable to tolerate cruelty. She was also prudent and truthful—"never misleads or misrepresents, however great the temptation." She attended her Catholic church regularly throughout life, which reinforced these inclinations.

Linda's early religious leanings were evident from her response to Dr. Terman's early questions about reading. In 1922 he presented a list of twenty-eight different types of readings. The children were requested to place an X in front of those they liked and two Xs in front of those they liked "very much." Although Linda placed Xs on twelve different lines, only three received double Xs: love stories, garden books, and the Bible. Religious reading found its place in her top three again in 1927. In adulthood many of Linda's health behaviors were consistent with what we know to be true of religious folks in general: she never smoked and she never drank alcohol. She remained an active member of her congregation, and so did her husband.

Although John and Linda shared some of the same childhood characteristics (he was described as "truthful, honest, and frank" as well as being more tender and sympathetic than the typical child), his lack of religious inclination was as clear as Linda's predisposition toward it. As a child and young adult, he rarely attended religious services and while in 1922 he marked twenty-five of the twenty-eight types of reading as enjoyable, he did not put an X on the line next to the Bible.

Donna fell in between the two—she didn't particularly care about reading the Bible, but as a teenager she listed religious reading as one of her preferred genres. Her church attendance during childhood was not as regular as Linda's, but her religious involvement increased over time, peaked in midlife, and then clearly tapered off after her sons left home.

We then asked ourselves: Was religious involvement at midlife predictive of long life during the ensuing decades? Before we get to those results, take a moment to reflect on your own religious experience.

SELF-ASSESSMENT: RELIGIOSITY

Answer each of the questions below as accurately as you can—some of these are exactly the same questions Dr. Terman asked his participants decades ago.

	Not at all 1 2 3 4 5 Very much
1. To what extent are you religiously inclined?	1 2 3 4 5
2. How much do you enjoy reading religious texts?	1 2 3 4 5
3. How regularly do you attend religious services?	1 2 3 4 5
4. How much do you pray?	1 2 3 4 5
5. How often do you watch religious programs on television or listen to them on the radio?	1 2 3 4 5
6. How involved are you with your religious community?	1 2 3 4 5

To calculate your score, simply add up your responses. Your result should fall between 6 and 30. Higher scores correspond with greater religiosity, but how should this be interpreted? It's not what you might first think. Having a low score is no reason for health panic and a high score is no assurance of long life because, as we discovered, not all elements of religiosity are equally important. We need to separate out the elements of being "religious" in order to understand how religion is relevant to health.

When we looked at whether religious involvement at midlife was predictive of long life during the ensuing decades, we saw that religiosity did not matter much for the men, a finding that has also surfaced in shorter-term studies by other researchers. But for the women, the religiously inclined were clearly more likely to live long lives.

In childhood these women tended to be more prudent, generous, and unselfish than the typical child. When they were teenagers, their parents described them as especially full of tenderness and sympathy and as having affectionate relations with their families. They grew up happier but somewhat more likely to conform to the authority of others, and they were optimistic about the future. They were, of course, less likely to smoke, abuse alcohol, and take illegal drugs. Importantly, in addition to being religious, these women tended to be socially involved and outgoing.

Trajectories of the Religious Women Who Lived Long

For the individual, of course, religiosity and religious attendance are not static and unchanging. Some people are and stay devout, others drift away, and still others become more devoted and spiritual over time. To understand the story in a way that included the importance of changes in religiousness over time, we teamed up with Professor Michael McCullough.[78] Mike has a well-deserved reputation for his research on revenge, forgiveness, and other such fascinating aspects of religion and health. Our measures of how religious each Terman subject was came from various questions they answered throughout many years. In addition to queries about the extent to which they were religiously inclined, they reported on their religious instruction, their Bible reading, their worship, and more. In our research, their answers were judged on religiosity, ranging from absolutely no religious interest to having a very strong religious inclination and involvement, at various points in time.

We again analyzed who lived the longest, now looking more fully at their life paths across the decades. Could it be that the long-lived women achieved an inner peace and self-healing through their long-term prayer and devotion? Which of their characteristics mattered most to long life?

The very religious women tended to be very friendly but were also inclined to be worriers. We found that we could explain their long lives by taking into account their outgoing yet concerned personalities, and their good, helpful social ties and behaviors, as they were measured in midlife. In other words, for these women, religion was a core and stable part of who they were and how they behaved—and it served them well in terms of long life.

It was the least religious women who were least likely to live a very long life. These women were not religious in young adulthood and stayed that way throughout their lives. They were generally bright and productive but they were less likely to be very extroverted and trusting, less likely to get and stay married, and less likely to have children or to be extensively involved in helping others.

What about the women like Donna whose religious inclinations declined with age? For them, we had to consider the various influences in their lives that occurred after 1940, as they aged. These women tended to be married, with children, and they, too, were careful about their health and often involved in volunteer service activities. As these women became less involved with religion, however, what emerged as important to their longevity were their social ties and health behaviors. Following her divorce, Donna was working hard to support her two boys, was disappointed in relationships, and had little time for or interest in friends and outside activities. In contrast to those who thrived, she had no strong social ties to replace the ones she lost as she gradually withdrew from church. Of course, the fact that she smoked with her associates at work also likely played a key role in her early death.

Herein lay the core of our striking finding: overall it was not religious involvement per se that was so important to long life, although it helped many women. Rather it was the other characteristics that tended to go along with being religious that explained why these women lived longer. It was not the meditative effect of prayer or the act of regular attendance at religious services that mattered. It was a much broader collection of associated acts and attributes. Those who gradually left their religious involvement were at high risk *if* they also let their community involvement falter and diminish.

If these findings about religious inclination and long life are not a fluke, then other well-designed studies should yield similar results. One seven-year health study examined the religious involvement of over ninety thousand American women aged fifty and older as part of the Women's Health Initiative.[79] This huge study did confirm that the women who were more religiously involved were less likely to die during the period of the study. This result remained even after taking into account influences such as age, ethnicity, income, education, and certain aspects of health status such as smoking and drinking. These confirming results, as well as those from other recent studies, increased our confidence that the detailed findings that have emerged from our studies of the Terman participants are pointing to some fundamental insights about the paths to good health.

What It Means for You: Guideposts to Health and Long Life

While we cannot provide empirical corroboration about whether being pious is important to gaining eternal life, we did uncover good evidence that at least some aspects of congregational participation are relevant to the length of one's present life. The guideposts we identified, however, do not point directly to the church, the synagogue, or the mosque. Nor do they steer us directly to the meditation garden, with incense and candles. Instead, the most important characteristics, especially for women, are linked to social networks and community engagement.

Look again at the questions you answered about your religious experience in this chapter, but now think not of your overall score but instead of *how* you got that score. Our findings suggest that someone who scores lots of points from feeling religious or from watching television evangelists will not likely have the same experiences, or positive outcomes, as someone who is actively engaged in a religious community.

For the Terman men, and often for men more generally, the relevance of religion to health is overwhelmed by other influences—their families and their careers. The Terman men relied more on their wives in social realms, and so religious ties were less important to their health. And those unmarried but healthy men like John, who was not at all religious in the traditional sense yet still lived a long life, usually maintained close relationships with friends and colleagues outside the context of religious organizations.

Some people feel they are not devout enough, and they resolve to meditate further or to spend more hours in prayer. While this makes many people feel better and more compassionate, our findings suggest that these practices are not central to health promotion. Instead, the good health habits fostered by religious practice and especially the social engagement that is so much a part of religious community are the likely explanations for the health of many religious folks.

After making this discovery, we needed to understand more about the social ties that appeared health promoting. Was it the secure feeling of being in a congregation or the volunteer work or having many friends? What steps can we take? We explore these matters, and the sometimes paradoxical discoveries, in the next chapter.

· CHAPTER 12 ·

Confidants, Networks, and the Power of Social Life

L inda had a lot of social connections, including with six other women she was in contact with weekly. Not only that, but her large extended family lived in the same town, fairly close to her home. James, in contrast, had fewer connections and associates, but he felt especially socially secure and supported. He perceived he could count on his now-adult offspring and he could confide in them whenever he wished. Many other sorts of social links were also apparent among the Terman participants. We wondered which aspects of social ties would be most relevant to health and long life.

Social support is a catchall phrase used to describe the ties we have to others. But it is too broad and confusing. Sometimes it refers to the size of your social network—how many friends and relatives you have, particularly how many you regularly see or talk to. At other times, researchers define social support as the feelings you have about being cared for—whether you have people who love you and cheer you up when you are down.

To confuse matters even further, sometimes researchers focus on the social support that comes from assisting others—measuring whether people come to you for advice and how often you lend a hand to friends and neighbors. Helping others, expressing gratitude, and acting as a mentor are healthy patterns that are often recommended to those trying to fight depression or improve their sense of well-being. These are well-known to work—to cheer you up—in the short term. But are they relevant to long life?

Our first challenge was to figure out how best to measure the social support of the Terman participants. While many researchers have conducted short-term studies of social support, they've used modern measures not available in Terman's time.

Combing the archives, with lots of help from graduate student Keiko Taga, we deemed certain activities and relationships to be markers of social support: frequency of visiting and communicating with relatives, friends, and neighbors; helping friends or neighbors; doing community service; satisfaction with friendships and social contacts; number of intimate and companionate relationships; quality relationships with family and close relatives; and frequency of meetings with social or community groups. Using statistical analyses, we combined and condensed this and other related information to reflect the major ways of viewing social support. In particular, we considered network size, feeling connected, and helping others. We then checked to make sure that our measures captured social support in the same way that modern measures do (using the same correlational approach we'd used for the personality scales).

SELF-ASSESSMENT: SOCIAL SUPPORT NETWORK

Answer each of the questions with your best estimate or assessment.

1. How often in a typical month do you talk to a lot of different people at parties?

   Never
   1
   2
   3
   4 or more times

2. How often in the past month have you participated in group meetings or activities (other than work meetings)?

Never
1
2
3
4 or more times

3. Of your friends, how many could you definitely call on for help if you needed it?

None
1
2
3
4 or more

4. How many relatives do you see or hear from at least once per month?

None
1
2
3
4 or more

5. How many people in your life accept you totally, just as you are?

None
1
2
3
4 or more

6. How often in the past month have friends or relatives made you feel loved and cared for?

Never
1
2
3
4 or more times

7. How many people can you count on to help you feel better when you are down in the dumps?

None
1
2
3
4 or more

8. How often in the past month have others   Never
   talked to you about important decisions they   1
   need to make?   2
                                                  3
                                                  4 or more times

9. How often in the past week have you helped   None
   others (beyond your partner or children) with 1
   tasks they needed to do?   2
                                                  3
                                                  4 or more times

10. How many people—including your children,   None
    parents, friends, and neighbors—rely on you   1
    to do something important for them every   2
    day?   3
                                                  4 or more

To calculate your overall score, ignore your answer to question 1, which is an irrelevant filler item, and add up your scores for questions 2 through 10. (Give yourself a 0 for each "none" or "never" response you circled, and a 4 for each "4 or more.") The total will fall somewhere between 0 (never/none) and 36. Although people vary widely in both social network size and their perceptions of how beneficial their social support networks are, we don't expect anyone to score a 0 on this scale. In fact, scoring below 7 is very unusual. Most people score at least in the double digits, and higher numbers (such as above 25) represent the strong social support that serves to promote longevity. But even more important than your overall score is your score on three subscales.

As we will see, items 2, 3, and 4 together assess the most important element, namely whether you have a large social network. Items 8, 9, and 10 assess the next important element, whether you help and provide support for others. Items 5, 6, and 7 assess the least important aspect of social support—whether you feel that others are there for you. In fact, we found that this last factor is overrated in terms of its health value. Feelings were not the key.

Social Butterflies

As we noted, Linda had a large social network. With her extended family nearby, she saw most of her relatives at least once a month. She also had a lot of friends. She saw two of these friends regularly in her congregation, and she talked to four other friends about health and career matters.

James felt socially secure and supported—perceiving that he could count on his now-grown children to help with daily tasks when needed. He felt they were genuinely interested in listening to him. He had some close friends with whom he would play cards, especially when he was worried or facing an important decision. In contrast to James, John's friendships tended to center around his career, though he did keep in touch with his wartime buddies.

Barbara, the social worker and overall humanist, had a different kind of social support—that which comes from helping others. She had good social relations not only because her job involved connecting to others, but because she also frequently assisted her friends and her church in organizing community service projects. What she loved most about her congregation was that it gave her the chance to help her friends and neighbors directly, as well as to reach out to those in need beyond her immediate social circle. We were now getting at the heart of the question to which our religion findings had pointed us: What aspects of social support matter most when it comes to longevity? Which pieces of congregational connections are most relevant to long life?

Social Support and Long Life

To determine which aspects of social ties were prominent on the path to long life, we examined how the various aspects of social support at around retirement age were related to mortality risk over the ensuing two decades. We figured that if a Terman participant sincerely felt that he or she had friends and relatives to count on when having a hard time then that person would be healthier. Those who felt very loved and cared for, we predicted, would live the longest. Surprise: our prediction was wrong. Although other studies have shown that people who feel loved and cared for will report a better sense of well-being—they *feel better*—we did not find that it helped much for living a long life.

What about focusing on the size of social networks rather than emphasizing only feelings? Does having regular contact with a large number of close, comfortable friends make a difference? A clear finding was that those who had a large social network lived longer. Just as we had seen in our studies of religiosity, social networks matter a lot.

Beyond social network size, the clearest benefit of social relationships came from helping others. Those who helped their friends and neighbors, advising and caring for others, tended to live to old age. Those like Barbara, who had large networks *and* good social relations because they helped others, were reaping a real benefit in terms of their longevity.[80]

Do the Good Die Young?

Over three hundred years ago Daniel Defoe, famous for his novel *Robinson Crusoe*, asserted, "The best of men cannot suspend their fate: The good die early, and the bad die late."[81] We did not find this to be true at all, instead finding that many of the most agreeable, thoughtful, and helpful Terman subjects, including Linda, were among the longest living.

That said, we saw again and again that it was not the feel-good aspects of having friends that was associated with long life. Rather, it was the more hands-on pieces that mattered most—being in contact with family members, doing things with friends, and helping others. When taken in total with the many other characteristics of long life—being conscientious, being in a good marriage, having healthy habits, and working hard in a successful career—Defoe's adage really crumbles. While his catchy saying has become a truism, repeated endlessly over the years in movies, songs, and philosophies, there's no real evidence that the good die young. In fact, although there are always some exceptions (which are therefore notable), generally speaking, it's the good ones who can actually help shape their fate; the bad die early, and the good do great.

Are Pets Truly Substitute Friends?

Animals often provide their owners with love, purpose, and security. Some researchers even suggest that pets are a good substitute for human companionship. It's true that animals can encourage healthy behaviors—when you take your dog for a daily walk, you are also getting a walk. And they encourage a degree of responsibility and organization. As pet owners and fans, we weren't about to argue a broad case against the benefits of having pets, but, over the long term, we wanted to see whether regularly interacting with pets produced measureable health benefits for the Terman participants.

In 1977, when they were in their sixties, the subjects were asked how often they played with pets—"never," "seldom," "occasionally," or "frequently." This was the perfect question, because we didn't care if someone had a pet but never interacted with that pet.

Using this question and the long life data, we looked to see whether those who played more with pets were more likely to survive over the next fourteen years. Another surprise: they were not. Not at all.[82]

Perhaps many of these pet aficionados already had good social support from people, meaning that animal companionship had little to add. If this were true, playing with pets would not be important for the group as a whole, but it might be quite important for those who were socially isolated. For them, pets could be filling in the gap that would otherwise be filled with people. We ran the statistical analyses again, this time looking just at the socially isolated. But the results were the same. Playing with pets wasn't associated with longer life.

We had to conclude that urging your elderly aunt who really doesn't like animals to get a dog so she will have a health-promoting companion is probably not a worthwhile idea. Having a pet is great if it brings joy to your life, but we found no evidence that it will provide the social enrichment that is so important to long life.

Social Life and Misconceptions about Life Expectancy

The average life expectancy of an American born around the time of the Terman participants (about 1910) was forty-seven years. The average life expectancy of an American born in recent years is about seventy-nine. Still, it is totally incorrect to conclude that today's middle-aged adults will live many, many years longer in retirement than did their predecessors.

The error arises from the fact that average life expectancy is computed from birth. For the Terman subjects' generation, many children died at birth or shortly thereafter. Many others died of childhood diseases. The twentieth century saw tremendous advances in sanitation, housing, food supply, and vaccines, leading to a dramatic plunge in deaths during infancy and childhood. So-called modern medical cures have played a relatively minor role in increasing adult life span, something most people do not understand.

The truth is that the life expectancy of a sixty-year-old white American male has only increased by about four or five years during the last half century, and some of that is likewise due to better housing, nutrition, safety (such as seat belts), and sanitation. It is a great misconception (with serious implications) in our society that modern medicine has led to huge increases in the longevity of American adults.

This distinction is important for understanding and appreciating the significance of social support and healthy life pathways. The Terman subjects on healthy life paths, with great social networks, were much more likely to live into their seventies, eighties, and nineties, while their fellow participants (who were equally healthy and intelligent as children, but didn't travel such healthy pathways) often succumbed before age sixty-five. The best surgical procedures and the most powerful pharmaceuticals of today are considered very successful if they extend life for several years. Of course if you are one of those patients, you are very grateful, but think of the much greater benefits that healthy pathways often produce—perhaps the decades of longer life that earlier sanitation advances, childhood vaccines, and public health measures achieved.

What It Means for You: Guideposts to Health and Long Life

The lives of the Terman participants showed that taking time to cultivate social networks is important not just to the quality of life but also to its quantity. Feeling good, staying calm, and breathing deeply can be signs of health but they are not its root causes. Instead, social relations should be the first place to look for improving health and longevity.

You may recall from the last chapter that John was not a religious person. Yet he lived a long life, and his social ties were a big part of his secret. For John, becoming more religious would not likely have improved his longevity because he was already enjoying the strongest benefits of being religious—the social elements. In contrast, Donna's case is one where congregational life could have made a huge difference. Donna didn't spend much time with friends or colleagues, focusing instead on raising her sons and just getting by after her divorce. When her sons were grown Donna pretty much quit going to church and became even more socially isolated. If Donna had instead become more involved in her church (or some other meaningful organizations), using her considerable intelligence to join with others to make a difference in her community, it very well might have improved her prospects for a long life.

John and Barbara found social connections in their careers. Barbara maintained additional social links through her congregation and extended network of friends. Linda's ties were mostly through family and church groups, but the effect remained the same. It was not those who *felt* the most connected and appreciated, but those who had many actual ties in their social networks, and who were engaged with helping others, who lived longest.

It is worth reiterating that social networks represent an important— perhaps the most important—way to change one's life pathway. In many ways, it is also a very doable fix, in a relatively straightforward manner. Repairing a troubled marriage or unproductive career is also very important to health but is quite difficult and will take a lot of time. In contrast, setting aside a few hours each week to volunteer, or joining a group that shares one of your passions, increases the size of your social network and provides opportunities to help others. You're never too old and it's never too late or too early to start this—and the returns can be enormous in terms of life's quality *and* quantity.

· CHAPTER 13 ·

The Gender Gap in Long Life

Almost everywhere in the world, women outlive men. This fact is so well appreciated that it figured in the long-running joke of the comedian Alan King: "Do you know the six words that appear in every man's obituary? *He is survived by his wife.*"

Perhaps fittingly, Mr. King himself was survived by his wife of fifty-seven years, Jeanette. Yet although this female advantage in longevity has long been studied, it remains puzzling. Many things contribute to this mysterious phenomenon, and not always in intuitive ways. For example, women generally face more health problems during their lives, yet men die earlier of most major causes of death, including heart disease, cancer, and suicide. While examining the pathways of the Terman participants we uncovered many fascinating hints as to why the average woman outlives the average man.

Possibly most intriguing is the relationship between the deaths of males and the deaths of their female spouses. The film director Edward Dmytryk, who died at ninety after a life full of challenges, was survived by his wife of sixty-four years. Norris Bradbury, the award-winning atomic physicist who lived to eighty-eight, was survived by his wife of almost sixty-five years. Even Ancel Keys, the cholesterol expert who lived to be a hundred was—yes—survived by his wife. However, what about those men who lost their wives? Many of the Terman men who were widowed did not live much longer after their loss. This was even the case for Terman himself—his wife, Anna Belle Minton Terman, died in early 1956, and he died later that same year, right before Christmas.

We know that much of the health and long life of the Terman men was facilitated by having a supportive wife and stable marriage, but was this related to the feminine dimensions typically provided by the wives? Did each spouse's masculinity/femininity and related traits really matter?

Measuring Masculinity and Femininity

Paul was a tough, masculine guy while James was more of a "family man." Linda was quite feminine while Donna was more of a tomboy. When we started investigating male-female differences in longevity we decided to distinguish biology from psychology—what is usually called the difference between biological sex and social gender. Biological sex refers to whether one is female or male—in chromosomal terms, XX or XY. Gender, on the other hand, refers to the psychosocial category of male-typical versus female-typical identities and behaviors. These are the qualities of masculinity versus femininity. You can easily relate to this difference by calling to mind girls who are labeled "girly girls" as compared to tomboys or contrasting a polite, "man of the arts" type with a rugged and somewhat crude "tough guy" type.

Being more masculine or feminine is not at all the same as being homosexual or heterosexual. Dr. Terman himself, more than a half century ago, explained it this way: "It would be a grave error to assume that any M-F [masculine-feminine] score approaching the mean of the opposite sex justifies in itself a diagnosis of homosexuality. One may be a fairly pronounced invert in sex temperament without being at all a sex invert [gay] in the usual sense."[83]

By the way, there were of course gays and lesbians in the study, and some married (the opposite sex), which was not unusual in the 1930s and 1940s. But because of the significant threats to individuals who were openly gay, Dr. Terman hid their identities. He even destroyed letters and other information. So our analyses of men and women could not directly take sexual orientation into account.

This issue of masculinity and femininity was a tricky subject to try to investigate. If we used typically male-associated behaviors like drinking, smoking, and promiscuity to define masculinity, then we would be biasing our results because these behaviors are known to be unhealthy. We had to find a way to evaluate masculinity and femininity without tapping into unhealthy lifestyles in our measures.

So we turned to a collaboration with well-known gender expert Dr. Richard Lippa at the California State University in Fullerton. Richard created "gender diagnosticity" scores indicating how masculine or feminine each person was. His approach is important because many traditional masculinity measures seem really to be measuring instrumentality—the quality related to serving a purpose and reaching a goal. In western cultures, instrumentality is more prevalent in men, for a variety of reasons. Many femininity scales seem really to be measuring emotionality or expressiveness—qualities of being caring and sensitive to others' feelings. Expressiveness is more prevalent in women. Although such masculinity and femininity scales are pretty good at describing the stereotypical man or woman, they aren't very good at taking account of certain other aspects of our understanding of what it means to be "masculine" and "feminine." More than that, they do not yield a good enough sense of health-relevant hobbies, interests, activities, and behaviors. And, importantly, we wanted to know how masculine or feminine each individual Terman participant was compared to his or her fellow subjects.

To create our gender diagnosticity scores, we went beyond the traditional measures, using information that Linda, Donna, James, Paul, and the others provided (at around age thirty) about their preferences and interests in various types of occupations. The participants had rated their degree of preference—like, indifference, or dislike—for about a hundred occupations. We then used statistical techniques to calculate gender diagnosticity scores from these preference ratings. Working backward, in order to avoid stereotypes, we computed the probability that a participant was male or female, given his or her occupational preferences. Mechanical engineer, factory manager, and chemist were male-type occupations, preferred by the Terman men. Interior decorator, florist, social worker, and librarian were female-type occupations, generally preferred by the women. By working in reverse, we were able to discover the masculine men and the more feminine men, as well as the more masculine women and the feminine women. And we were able to avoid stereotypes. Who lived the longest?

Masculine and Feminine Men

Paul (the sardonic jokester), predictably, scored as highly masculine—he gave higher preference ratings to the occupations that other Terman men chose, and gave low interest ratings to the occupations that were typically chosen by women. Outgoing and something of a loudmouth, Paul was a classic "man's man." Although his career path took him in various directions, not all of them stereotypically masculine (recall that he drifted from newspaper reporter to salesman, proofreader, and finally bookstore manager), his interests and identity were far from feminine. He was an active child, reported by his mother as having an "extraordinary amount of physical energy, 'pep' and animation. Dynamic and tireless." He was curious and mischievous, which sometimes got him into trouble. Though he didn't suffer any serious accidents in childhood, he had a lot of skinned knees. His mother also noted that he was punished "rather frequently" and that physical punishment seemed to work best. An avid sports fan, both as a participant and a spectator, Paul played shortstop on baseball teams from the time he was in third grade until he finished college. He also played intramural football throughout his college years and was a supporter of the local sports teams. His other hobbies included sportswriting, camping, hunting, electronic gadgetry, and sports cars.

The ever-tactful James, in contrast, was lower on the masculinity scale. A thoughtful husband to his wife, Irene, and involved father to his three children, the sensitivity James's mother had noted many years earlier ("sensitive to approval or disapproval of other children. Can't endure to be disliked") had developed into something more akin to empathy. Rather vain as a child (he was described in elementary school as one who "fishes for praise"), his awareness of the perceptions of others probably helped him to excel later in his job as a public relations officer. Though of average musical talent, James enjoyed music, and he demonstrated an extraordinary appreciation for beautiful colors and forms; his mother noted that at an early age he had "natural taste." Original and resourceful in childhood, James was described as a nonconformist by his wife, and indeed his hobbies failed to conform to traditional male stereotypes—he listed art, movies, music, and attending plays as his favorite pastimes. All told, James scored fairly high on femininity, showing more interest in the occupations that women tended to choose than Paul had.

Masculine and Feminine Women

Donna, who as a child enjoyed playing marbles, watching sports, and collecting arrowheads, moved easily in a traditional man's world. She smoked, she did not hesitate to drink, and she competed well on the job. Unlike many women of her generation, she didn't keep quiet. When we computed her likes and dislikes, Donna scored quite high on masculinity, though not as high as Paul; she showed a good deal of interest in and preference for jobs that Terman men had tended to prefer.

In contrast with Donna, whose interests and activities earned her the reputation of a "romp," Linda, who married when she was twenty, was anything but a tomboy. Her interests centered around homemaking and her children. Although she enjoyed socializing, her family was at the top of her priority list. Giving to a fault (her parents, in fact, described her as "too generous" in 1936), she was also somewhat sensitive, and she indicated in her self-evaluation that her feelings could be easily hurt. Fortunately, she and her husband only occasionally disagreed, communicating well as they planned the family budget, made

arrangements together for holidays, confided their worries to one another, and exchanged jokes.

Linda was highly feminine, choosing occupations that most other
women also endorsed as the most desirable. James, who also scored
fairly high on femininity, did not score as high as Linda—he showed
more interest in the occupations that women tended to choose than
Paul did, but not as much interest in those jobs as Linda did.

SELF-ASSESSMENT: MASCULINITY AND FEMININITY

*If you were free to pursue any occupation you desired (that is, if the
length of time you'd need to be in school or the cost of tuition were not
factors to be considered), what would you choose? What are you passionate about? Which hobbies or jobs would you find wholly unappeal-
ing? On the list below, assign a number to each of the seventeen types
of jobs and activities in accordance with your preferences.*

Occupation/ Activity	-2: I would really hate it	-1: It wouldn't be too bad	0: I could take it or leave it	+1: I would like it okay	+2: I would really love it
College professor					
Mechanical engineer					
Interior decorator					
Watching figure skating					
Athletic director					

Landscape gardener					
Hearing about other people's problems					
Interpreter					
Pilot					
Physician					
Bank teller					
Social worker					
Bookkeeper					
Playing competitive sports					
Novelist					
Inventor					
Working with children					

To compute your score, first cross off physician, bank teller, and bookkeeper. Terman men and women were equally likely to endorse these occupations—they are neither "masculine" nor "feminine." College professor and novelist were slightly correlated with gender in our sample—men were a little more likely to endorse professor and women to endorse novelist (but not by much). So cross those off, too. Now, for interior decorator (the most "feminine" occupation listed), social worker, interpreter, working with children, hearing about other people's problems, watching figure skating, and landscape gardener, reverse your scores. That is, change your minus to plus (or plus to minus); if you marked 0 leave it as it is. Mechanical engineer is the most "masculine" occupation on this list; it is followed by inventor, pilot, athletic director, and playing competitive sports. For these, do not make any changes to your score. Now, simply add up your total.

The most masculine score is +24, while the most feminine is −24. Although there are various limits in this type of assessment, preferences for the occupations and leisure activities that are listed can give some idea about how masculine or feminine you are, in terms relevant to understanding the Terman participants. To give you a contemporary comparison, college students at the lowest quartile (more feminine) today score about -12 while those at the highest quartile are at +15 (more masculine).

Times have changed and with them the gender roles and norms associated with jobs, hobbies, and so on. Among the Terman subjects, women indicated stronger interest in landscape gardening than did men, although today it might be a more male-typical activity. This is a good example of how details about gender roles and concepts of what is masculine or feminine are shaped in part by society (including the media) and influenced by people's changing behaviors. But some people still gravitate to one side of the activity spectrum while others move toward the other side. Details evolve over time, but the principles remain the same.

Femininity and Long Life

Among men, the more masculine tended to be heavier, more physically active, and to have riskier hobbies. Among women, the more masculine tended to drink more and earn more money. That made sense, but the question remained: Who lived longer?

The eye-opener in our findings was that the more masculine men *and* the more masculine women had an increased mortality risk, while the more feminine women *and* the more feminine men were relatively protected. It seems that part of what helps women to live longer isn't just that they're female, but the fact that women are, on average, more feminine than men.[84]

In other words, the gender gap in longevity isn't all based on the Y chromosome. Those who skewed more feminine—women like Linda and men like James—often had similar mortality risks, whereas those who were more masculine—like Paul and Donna—were also somewhat alike.

What is it that makes femininity a helpful characteristic, at least in terms of the length of life? Some of it has to do with gender roles—that is, the things that society says are appropriate for men versus women to do. For example, it used to be quite common for men to smoke but rather uncommon for women (especially feminine women) to do so. This changed in the 1970s, as illustrated by cigarette advertisements for Virginia Slims, which were specifically marketed to women: "You've come a long way, baby!" And when it did, women's mortality risk and cancer risk rose. When smoking, a behavior that seriously threatens health, was primarily carried out by men, with only the more adventurous, less feminine women daring to light up, men as a group had a much greater likelihood of dying from various cancers and other smoking-related causes than women. As women's roles changed, and smoking became an acceptably feminine behavior, the difference in risk from smoking-related causes began to narrow. Though important, that finding itself is not very surprising.

But smoking is only part of the story. When we analyzed causes of death, we found that feminine women and feminine men were less likely to die from *all* causes, not just cancer or smoking-related diseases.

As ideas about men and women have changed, we wondered if this masculine-feminine difference was confirmed by health statistics from recent decades. As one example, in the Terman years, when men held primary financial responsibility for the family and were working in more hostile environments than were most women, the rate of cardiovascular disease was significantly higher for men than for women. Women's lives, on the contrary, often centered around the home and neighborhood—a more "feminine" environment. However, as women entered the workplace in greater numbers—frequently taking on many traditionally masculine responsibilities—some men moved in the opposite direction—taking on more social and emotional roles—and another bit of the male-female difference in lifelong mortality risk (including cardiovascular risk) disappeared.[85] It is entirely possible, by our reading, that these mortality shifts are related to the changes in masculinity and femininity, in men and women.

Social Ties and Gender

Perhaps the issue wasn't stress, but coping. Among the Terman children, being moody in childhood was relevant to increased mortality risk for boys but not for girls.[86] Similarly, later in life it was the Terman men who had experienced mental difficulties and breakdowns who were at greatest risk for earlier mortality.[87] Stereotypes would suggest that these men were coping by using typically masculine unhealthy mechanisms like heading out to the bar. It turned out, however, that differences in coping with stress through smoking and drinking alcohol did not explain the mortality discrepancies.

What did masculine and feminine personalities dictate in terms of social ties? The idea was that moody women or those struggling with mental health issues might be better able to garner resources by letting others know about their problems. In general, women report more symptoms of ill health (both physical and mental), seek more care than do men, and are more ready to admit when they need help.[88] Masculine men, on the other hand, may be especially unwilling to admit weakness or to seek help. In looking at the data, we confirmed that those who demonstrated male-typical characteristics were less outgoing and sociable and had weaker social support networks. The most masculine tended to keep others at an emotional distance. So we wondered what happened to masculine men after they lost their partners.

Men's Health After Loss

What happens to men, especially masculine men, when their wives die, breaking their key social support lifeline? As we saw earlier in this book, a stable and healthy marriage can indeed nudge one toward long life while the stresses associated with divorce are health harming. We also saw that the effects of divorce were dramatically different for men and women—men suffered more ill effects than did women. Might it be that women and men would also adjust differently to the death of their life partner? And would the personality characteristics of the surviving spouse be relevant?

Although various scientific studies suggest that a man's risk of dying can increase after the death of his spouse, the reasons why this occurs are not fully established. Sometimes the men seem to die of a "broken heart"—without a close social tie, they simply lose the will to live. In other cases, the wife was an important regulator of health behaviors, and without her reminders and encouragement, the bereaved man fails to take care of his health. So we were curious to know which characteristics allowed some widowers to thrive anyway.

How did men's and women's experience of widowhood differ, and might personality influence the reactions to bereavement? Most studies of the effects of bereavement are limited because they begin after the bereavement or, occasionally, right before. In other words, if you were going to study the effects of the death of one's partner, you would start by finding people who had lost their spouses (or were about to). This is common sense but it is inadequate in a scientific sense for two reasons: a person's characteristics can change during bereavement, and the appropriate comparison groups—of people not bereaved—are not included. No study had ever looked comprehensively at preexisting characteristics, such as personality, to see if they were related to how well people do after losing a spouse, compared to those who have not lost a spouse.

We went back to the measures of the Terman subjects' personalities using their responses in 1940, when they were about thirty years old, now limiting our focus to those who were married. We classified them according to whether they were widowed during the following four decades and then looked at how long they lived, over the next sixty-plus years.

Overall, of course, the women outlived the men. Not only that, but the widowed women tended to thrive—they lived longer than the still-married women. In fact, many widowed women went on to live exceptionally long lives.[89]

Not only were there differences between men and women; personality also mattered. The most surprising finding involved the sensitive, neurotic, worrying men. People generally don't strive to be neurotic. No one wants to seem overly anxious, worrying, and moody. And generally speaking, neuroticism isn't a trait that predisposed subjects to a long life. It held no magic at all for widowed women, as they turned their lives toward their friends and their children rather than worrying about themselves. But for widowed men, the picture was dramatically different. When men who had lost their wives were also highly neurotic, their subsequent mortality risk was reduced—by half![90]

For the married men who were not bereaved, their degree of neuroticism didn't impact their longevity. What could be going on here? It seems that the worriers were much more willing to take care of their health after their wives were gone. Generally speaking, the masculine man is less willing to get that prostate exam, put on the seat belt, complain to the doctor, or worry about blood pressure. This is especially a problem when his wife is gone. But being a worrier reduced these risks. In this narrow circumstance, worrying compensated for the dearth of social ties.

This explanation fits with the other things we know about men, marriage, and health. It certainly seemed to be the case for James, who lost his wife in 1987, a little after their golden anniversary. In middle adulthood he had described himself as somewhat moody and a worrier—a person who sometimes couldn't keep nagging thoughts from coming into his head to distract him. James was one of the widowers who lived on well past his wife's death. Somehow those neurotic, nagging thoughts and pinpricks of anxiety served James well, keeping him involved in his own health and extending his life.

This startling finding about neurotic men serves as a good reminder of just how complex the interactions are between internal characteristics (such as personality) and external factors (such as bereavement). Only looking at individual life paths over the long term allows us to properly understand these kinds of health threats and benefits.

What It Means for You: Guideposts to Health and Long Life

Women significantly outlive men, not only among the Terman participants but in almost any group. The reasons for this difference are complicated, and no one has yet fully explained them all. But our studies of the Terman men and women across the decades have yielded some tantalizing clues. Although the average man lives a shorter life than the average woman—five to seven years shorter—there is quite a bit of overlap and variation.

One might have guessed that the more masculine women, who got out and took charge of their lives, would have outlived the women who liked more traditional, home-based activities like interior decorating and working with children. But this was not what we found. One might also think that among the men, it would be the jocks and sports fans who stayed fit and lived long. But here again, that was not what happened across the decades. For most, femininity was more protective and masculinity was more dangerous.

James's nurturing of his more feminine side—for him, theater and music—led him to develop a great network of friends and a close family. Yes, he was sensitive and a worrier, but that helped him cope well with his challenges, including the death of his wife.

Overall, in various studies, we repeatedly discovered that the women would generally recover and thrive even if they lost their men, whether by divorce or widowhood. Longevity often seemed to come down to social relations. The women and the less masculine men were better able to establish and maintain deeper social connections, which often saved their lives.

Our use of data-derived notions of masculinity and femininity made it clear to us that it is an especially good idea to nurture one particular feminine quality: social connectedness. Over and over in our research we have seen the value of social networks. Healthy aging involves maintaining contact with family and community. Meaningful bonds with others are part of the reason that being active in one's religious congregation is healthy. A close, loving relationship with one's spouse promotes long life. And, in the case of those who endured parental divorce during childhood, establishing good social relations helps blunt the risk associated with that stressful experience.

In today's world the benefits of traditionally masculine qualities are obvious—those who are independent, aggressive go-getters tend to do well in their careers. The success they enjoy is something tangible and readily apparent. The benefits of traditionally feminine characteristics, however—especially being able to develop close social ties—are not always so easy to see. And yet it is precisely these qualities that buffer against life's hardships. Both men and women can often benefit from strengthening the interpersonal bonds that the more feminine people seem to find easier to nurture. And parents can help their children develop close ties by modeling empathic relationships in their own lives.

Such findings prompt a rethinking about one's personal characteristics and habits within particular situational contexts. Some believe they must be perfectionists, finding all the right behaviors and training themselves to do them; however this often results in feelings of exasperation when the "correct" personality characteristics don't come effortlessly. But we discovered that relevant strengths often appear unexpectedly. It is the lifelong developmental path, traveled by the self-aware individual who is willing to make thoughtful adjustments, that eventually has the highest chance of leading to long life. And more than that, certain personality traits and habits that you might think of as detrimental (such as being a worrier like James), once the tides have shifted, can become exactly the thing that keeps you alive. The Terman participants thus taught us that it is not always sensible to define a complex personality characteristic like neuroticism as "good" or "bad." The anxious, worrying moodiness that is less than ideal in some contexts was of benefit to men who lost their spouses and were left to fend for themselves.

Many fascinating aspects of gender, masculinity, and femininity remain unexplored. The adventurous, independent Shelley Smith Mydans, who was said to have had more stressful adventures than a soldier of fortune, lived a very long life but was survived by her husband. This case and several others like it raise an intriguing question: Does it matter not only how masculine or feminine you are, but also how masculine or feminine your partner is? Would a more masculine woman be healthier with a more masculine or more feminine partner? As far as we know, this question has never been seriously studied in this way.

· CHAPTER 14 ·

The Toll of War and Trauma

Why Some Thrive

In 1941 Philip became a soldier. Like about 350 of his fellow male Terman study participants, he served in the Second World War. About half of these men were mustered into the armed forces as privates, but many entered as officers. One became a brigadier general. Five of the participants were killed in the war, including one who was taken prisoner by the Japanese at Corregidor and died while being moved to a prison camp in China. But many more were *indirect* casualties, dying in later years partially as a result of their stressful wartime experiences.

Stress is often viewed as the boogeyman—the terrifying specter—of modern life. Watch out or it will get you! Yet many people face very challenging new circumstances, even war and terrorism, and do just fine. Many elderly veterans remember the awful pressures and traumas but thrive in good health. Why do others succumb? The astonishingly rich decades of data helped us to understand not only why many veterans thrived—but also why anyone who faces a traumatic challenge might very well be able to recover, prosper, and flourish.

Philip and many of the Terman men in the armed forces served in combat, but a significant number served in support roles. Some went overseas while others served in Washington, D.C., or on home bases. Many others contributed to the war effort in their civilian roles, especially as aircraft engineers, architects, chemists, and administrators, both inside and outside government. What they did and why they did it made a huge difference to their later health.

War and Stress

In Philip's case, the war cost him dearly. As a child in 1922, fidgety Philip was described as charismatic and a bit vain, not particularly diligent for a smart student, and somewhat prone to anxiety. He was not one of the more conscientious Terman children, but with his intelligence and engaging interpersonal style he got along well. After he married Arlene in 1935, he was quite content sharing their interests in music and social activities. They had a baby girl, Margaret. But despite his good health, loving family, and steady work, Philip remained uneasy, according to his parents. His own self-assessment in 1940 corroborated this, suggesting that his childhood tendencies toward neuroticism and low conscientiousness had carried through into adulthood. In their 1936 report, his parents noted Philip's apparent inability to save and be prudent with money, despite the tough economic times.

Philip joined the war effort and was soon a noncommissioned officer bound for the Aleutian Islands. By the time he returned home, in 1945, he had been swept far south and had seen combat in the Philippines, Guadalcanal, and the Solomon Islands. In addition to the stresses of combat, Philip felt the pain of the long separation from his wife and daughter. Shortly after his return, he reported feeling ambivalent about his wartime service. Although he realized that there were positive aspects to his service, he was frustrated and resentful over his circumstances and felt that both his child and his marriage had suffered as a result of his absence.

Philip and Arlene separated shortly after he returned from the Pacific, then reunited, then separated again. He felt that she "no longer cared" and that his time away had created an emotional distance between them. They were divorced in 1947. Philip remarried less than one year later. A light to moderate drinker before the war, Philip's alcohol use increased dramatically upon his return. Research studies have shown this to be generally true—men exposed to trauma or extreme stress are very likely to increase their drinking and, if available, their use of other drugs.

In 1950 Philip responded to a question about his use of liquor by remarking, "I am a fairly heavy drinker; I drink to excess rather frequently but do not feel that it has interfered seriously with my work or relationships with others." He stated that he still enjoyed music and was a member of the Chamber of Commerce, the Army and Navy Club, and the Elks.

In 1955 Philip reported having high blood pressure, insomnia, and congestive heart disease. By 1960 he listed more health problems, including "slight heart trouble" and angina. He was still engaged with the Army and Navy Club but indicated that his leisure time included "less physical activity." He also noted that his attempts to stop drinking had been unsuccessful. When asked what aspects of his life brought him the most satisfaction he listed his marriage as most important, and his children second.

Over the next decade Philip kept drinking, reported suffering from depression, and indicated that his heart disease was worsening. In 1972 he described his health as "fair" and said that he had to limit some of his activities due to low energy levels. He stated that his work was "tolerable" but said he would be glad to escape it when it was time to retire, which he believed would be in just a few years. He was looking forward to having time to "do more of the things [we] never had time to do." As he anticipated his retirement, he wasn't able to say that he expected to enjoy those years thoroughly; instead he said that he had "little idea what life will be like then." Philip didn't get a chance to find out. He died at age sixty-four from a massive heart attack.

Desk Jockeys vs. Infantrymen: The Effects of Stressful War Service

Over two hundred of the Terman men were sent overseas in the war, while about one hundred were stationed and remained in the United

States. To study the long-term effects of service in the armed forces, we teamed up with the distinguished sociologist Glen Elder and his colleagues Scott Brown and Elizabeth Clipp.[91] The team's research assistants, with knowledge of American military history, constructed records that documented the wartime experiences of each Terman study veteran.

After determining which of the servicemen went overseas, we analyzed whether they had faced combat. The combat experiences revealed in the records included being fired upon, witnessing death and destruction, and going missing or being taken prisoner. We also knew who had received Silver Stars and Purple Hearts.

We were not able, however, to ascertain the precise depth of combat each man faced. This means that our findings about the effects of war are underestimates, as some precision of measurement is missing. That is, things are probably even worse than what we found.

Looking at the risk of death during the half century following the end of the war, we discovered that the men who had served overseas were more than one and a half times as likely to die in any given year (after the war) than were those veterans who served only on the home front. That is, those who went overseas and survived their deployment were much more likely than their compatriots to become ill and pass away in the years after they returned home. Was it stress?

Where You Fight Your Battles

With Midway, the Marshall Islands, Peleliu, Iwo Jima, and more, the fighting in the Pacific was especially fierce, with sea battles, island warfare, and aircraft carrier–based air combat. So we zeroed in on fighting in this area. We asked whether duty in the Pacific theater of war—what Philip faced—produced different long-term consequences than did military service in Europe. Although the fight against the Nazis was certainly no picnic, the Pacific theater was especially brutal. Soldiers fighting in Asia faced tropical diseases, island-to-island fighting, distant cultures, and especially harsh enemy tactics.

In contrast to Philip, John spent three years doing intelligence work in England. Although his contribution was crucial to the war effort, and it entailed a good deal of stress, he didn't usually have to worry about his personal safety and he was able to maintain regular contact with his parents and siblings back in Palo Alto, California. Late in the war, he knew about and had to come to terms with Nazi atrocities in the concentration camps. Some of his associates landed at Normandy on D-day, but none of his close friends were killed in combat. He maintained ties with his wartime "buddies" after his return home, transitioning rather smoothly back into his civilian job and life.

In a series of statistical analyses, we found that those men like Philip who fought against the Japanese in the Pacific theater were much more likely to die during the ensuing five postwar decades than were those men like John who served elsewhere overseas. The theater of fighting made a difference.

When we looked at the postwar mortality risk for those men who were sent overseas *and* faced combat as compared to those who were sent overseas but did not face the stress of direct combat, a consistent picture began to emerge. The combat veterans were less likely to go on to live long lives. In a fascinating finding, each stress posed a distinct risk—serving overseas, serving in the Pacific, and facing combat. The more alien and disturbing the situation, the worse the later health.

Personality and Battle Roles: The Surprising Selection

As often happens in our Terman studies, an unanticipated twist appeared as we pored over the statistical analyses—a finding with ramifications even for those who will never put on a uniform. We had seen before that the lives and paths of the participants were much less random than they first appeared. Could this be true even for wartime experiences, which are so heavily shaped by the demands of the military? We knew that conscientiousness measured in childhood was highly relevant to a whole host of later-life health trajectories. Could it even be relevant to war?

Even we were surprised to discover that the more conscientious subjects, such as John, were less likely to be sent to the Pacific theater. That is, the more careless, vain, and impulsive a man had been as a child (like Philip), the more likely he was to wind up fighting the Japanese in very dangerous and stressful Pacific operations.

As a child, Philip was impetuous and full of energy. He had plenty of friends despite his bouts of moodiness and his attention-seeking behaviors. Throughout his life he seemed to have more health problems than the average Terman participant. Although none of these illnesses was particularly severe, every report mentioned physical ailments ranging from tonsillitis in childhood to an ulcer, fungus infection, and sinus problems in adulthood. Over the course of his adult life Philip's financial status fluctuated; on more than one occasion he reported to Dr. Terman that he had money worries.

Although sometimes a meteorlike strike would come out of nowhere and smack down a Terman participant, it was more often the case that an accumulation of small decisions and reactions would lead to large and significant consequences. While we have no direct information about why the less conscientious, like Philip, were more likely to end up serving in the Pacific, this fascinating discovery, taken in context with our other findings, leads to interesting conjectures about paths to long life: those traveling dangerous byways often crashed, and it repeatedly goes well beyond bad luck.

Most people who face serious trauma do not go on to face long-term problems or to be classified as suffering from post-traumatic stress disorder (PTSD). Sure, they may turn anxious in certain evocative situations or they may be more aware of the fragility of life, but most do not struggle with chronic nightmares, ongoing irritability, and disrupted social relations. But many do face PTSD, perhaps up to a third of trauma victims. As we revealed, such serious stress is a major threat to health.

Why Is Traumatic Stress Harmful?

Scientists know a lot about what happens inside a human body under stress, as the brain struggles to preserve the health of the body. Hormones are released as the body revs up to be able to fight an enemy, flee a threat, battle a germ invader, repair a wound, or cope with a loss. So in many ways, stress is a good thing. The problem arises when the body cannot settle back down and instead keeps revving—what is usually called chronic stress. It is almost as if the brakes have failed and the vehicle is in constant danger of careening out of control.

Nevertheless, we scientists have been much less successful at thinking about stress across the long term. One cannot and should not "stop stressing" as one might "stop smoking." In fact, the stress response is essential to staying healthy.

The lifelong Terman study allows us to look not only inside the body at disease, longevity, and cause of death, but also *outside* the body. That is, the lifetimes of remarkable data permit a look at how stress at one point causes a host of problems at later points.

The journeys of the Terman participants down different life pathways revealed a simple but powerful way to think about stress: health problems arise when you veer off a healthy pathway and cannot steer back to safety. For example, when Patricia's parents divorced and her world turned upside down, she needed to react and adapt. She didn't choose Donna's path, which included smoking and drinking. Instead, she stayed in school, kept her conscientious friends, and later established a good marriage and career for herself. She lived a long life. But for those like Donna, chronic stress can feed on itself, leading to more and more destructive patterns. In particular, those on long life paths paired their individual strengths with their good social relations to get back on a road to healthier patterns.

The same is true of more severe, traumatic stress. The Terman war veterans who encountered traumatic stress and died young drove off the road. Alcohol was one of the key later problems for those who had faced wartime combat. Consistent with other research, we found that these Terman men were more likely to develop drinking problems, which in turn raised their postwar risk of dying. Many, but not all, were also less likely to go back and conscientiously complete the advanced education toward which they were headed prior to leaving for war. Sadly, they were not only especially likely to die from diseases commonly associated with stress—heart disease and injuries or accidents. The stress-filled paths often took a toll throughout their bodies.

Depression and Heart Disease

A close companion of chronic stress—and a bad sign—is depression. This was the case with Philip, who suffered regular bouts of depression, never severe, but enough to be a concern. As a good deal of research now documents, the fact that he was chronically stressed and a catastrophizer made it likely that he would get depressed. And the fact that he was depressed made it much more likely that he would die of heart disease, and at a relatively young age. Depression is a risk factor for many illnesses but is an especially well-established risk factor for heart disease.

What is unclear in Philip's case—and for the many millions of others who battle depression—is whether or not the depression per se was the problem. This matter is one of the most important in all of health and health care, yet it is one in which we think there's a terrible degree of misunderstanding.

When the stress of war or trauma leads to severe depression and then to suicide, it is clear that depression has played a key causal role in the early death. An obvious intervention along the way would be to treat the depression. Of course this often works—individuals who come out of their depressed state have their risk of suicide fall dramatically.

The case of stress, depression, and heart disease is much more complicated, however. Back a number of years ago, one of us (Howard) and his student Stephanie Booth-Kewley did several quantitative reviews—meta-analyses—of relevant studies involving depression and disease. Surprisingly similar patterns appeared between a variety of psychological predictors like depression and multiple diseases. This contradicted the then-prevailing notions of a distinct type A "coronary-prone personality," a distinct "ulcer-prone personality," and so on.

This broader pattern—having a *disease-prone personality*—suggested that negative traits such as depression, and its complements—hostility and aggressiveness—are markers of increased risk for both cardiovascular disease and a host of other illnesses.[92] This conclusion has since been confirmed by others. No narrow coronary-prone personality was found—suggesting that perhaps some underlying variables were affecting both the likelihood of depression and the likelihood of heart disease. If that were true, then treating depression would not necessarily affect the risk of heart disease.

To find out, a large national study evaluated the role of depression in heart attacks.[93] Over two thousand men and women who had suffered a heart attack were enrolled in the study and followed, and any depression was assessed. Depression was then treated in half of the participants, with therapy and with antidepressive drugs when necessary. The rest of the patients received standard medical care. Did those who had their depression treated then live longer or have fewer other heart problems? Not at all! Treating depression had no effect on extending life or preventing another heart attack. Depression was not the *cause* of the ill health.

The Terman studies give us an insight as to what is likely going on here. Individuals who are depressed are on a pathway *associated* with poor health and increased risk of dying. Their depression comes from many places, causing many ripples—biological predisposition being one of them. Also contributing are unhealthy habits, a weakened capacity to cope with stress, and impaired social relations.

If this is the case, then the Terman subjects who were generally mentally healthier and better adjusted should live longer. We went back and re-created an index of psychological maladjustment through midlife that Dr. Terman and his colleagues had diagnosed as of 1950 (five years after World War II ended). Most were able to cope with the challenges of their lives. Others, however, felt inadequate or had shown significant symptoms of anxiety or depression, or had suffered a nervous breakdown. We then created a second index—our own measure of adjustment—based on the 1950 responses as to whether the subject was self-confident and content, could get along with others, was moody, felt inferior, and was sensitive and thin-skinned.

We computed the statistical analyses for predicting long life, and, sure enough, poorer mental health and less maturity in 1950 were related to higher risk of mortality over the half century that followed. This was especially true for the men. These were the individuals who, by their forties, had strayed off the healthier paths to long life, often pushed along by stressful wartime experiences. Not only were those who were not well-adjusted in 1950 at higher risk of dying from all causes, they were especially more likely to die from violence (including suicide) and cardiovascular disease.[94]

Where many clinicians and researchers go wrong is to think of depression as a risk factor like smoking. If you stop smoking, your disease risks start decreasing immediately. But depression is more like adult-onset diabetes or other disorders of metabolism—it is caused by and leads to many different things and cannot be simply, permanently cured. Instead, setting off on a healthier pathway is the way to slowly but surely improve both depression and other aspects of health.

If you or a friend or loved one is facing serious anxiety or depression in young adulthood, then this is not only a sign of possible short-term threats to well-being, such as eating disorders, drinking, drug abuse, driving accidents, and even suicide and other violence; it is also a warning of long-term disease threats to health. But the treatment focus should not only be on the severe anxiety and depression. Rather, a broader view is most valuable, in which the individual is slowly integrated back into a supportive community, a stable career, and a caring family or group of close friends. This is not easy to do, but when such folks get moving on this new path, the results are often remarkably deep, wide-ranging, and long lasting.

Women and War Trauma

As was the case with most American women during the war, few of the Terman women served directly. Only about a dozen were formally committed to the war effort—including four in the Women's Army Corps (WAC, the women's branch of the U.S. Army) and five in the navy's WAVES (Women Accepted for Volunteer Emergency Service). Many Terman study women were engaged in war-related work in the government, in industry, or in other crucial positions such as in the Red Cross or in potentially risky information-related positions (such as that of Shelley Smith Mydans, the *Life* magazine reporter who was captured by the Japanese in Manila). However, there was not enough information for us to evaluate later health effects of the women's war contributions and experiences.

SELF-ASSESSMENT: TRAUMATIC EXPERIENCES

Think about the most serious and traumatic events you have faced in your life, such as suffering a serious physical assault; facing military combat; being at or near the sites of the September 11 terrorist attacks or other major terrorist attacks; losing a very close friend or relative to suicide or murder; being raped or sexually or physically abused; or experiencing a major fire, flood, or similar major catastrophe. (If you are lucky enough to never have faced such a challenge, then you probably are not at risk from such stress.) Evaluate how much the following statements apply to you.

Not at all true of me   1 2 3 4 5 Very true of me

1. I always try to avoid thinking about my stressful
   experience.   1 2 3 4 5

2. I try to avoid all stressful events because they may
   set off my feelings about the stressful trauma.   1 2 3 4 5

3. Since the event, I cry easily or feel my heart
   pounding and my body sweating in the face of even
   minor disruptions.   1 2 3 4 5

4. I have given up planning for the future.   1 2 3 4 5

5. I have vivid, recurring nightmares.   1 2 3 4 5

6. I feel emotionally numb, cut off even from those
   close to me.   1 2 3 4 5

7. I get very upset when reminded of the trauma and
   avoid situations that are reminders.   1 2 3 4 5

8. I have (daytime) flashbacks of the event.   1 2 3 4 5

9. I have been diagnosed with depression, probably
   triggered from trauma or severe stress.   1 2 3 4 5

10. I have been diagnosed with
    post-traumatic stress disorder (PTSD).   1 2 3 4 5

Because this kind of severe stress can involve complicated psycho-logical reactions and be an immediate significant threat to your health in complex ways, we do not provide a scoring system for this scale. But clearly the higher your score, the greater the possibility that you are suffering from health-harming chronic stress. The items help us understand the psychological aspects of significant chronic stress, as opposed to usual, normal worrying. If you get the sense that many of these items apply to you or someone close to you, then professional intervention from a mental health professional is advisable. There are excellent treatments available.

Stress and Genes

Here's a dilemma. Many people are comfortable believing that stress and instability can cause health problems. Yet many of the same people think that health is mostly in the genes. We hear of certain hereditary diseases that are tightly tied to genetic makeup. For example, the pioneering American folk singer Woody Guthrie suffered from Huntington's disease. This is a genetic neurodegenerative disorder wherein defective inherited genes tell nerve cells to atrophy and die; if you have this genetic mutation you will develop this devastating condition. We also know that many common individual characteristics are heavily genetic: the tallest Terman subject was six feet nine inches tall, and not because he was calm and loved to drink orange juice. Many people thus assume that our health, like our height, depends mostly on our genetic luck. Which is true—stress or genes?

Both stress *and* genes are important, and this is not a hedge but rather a scientific finding. Most health threats in adulthood are not caused directly and simply by defective inherited genes. On the other hand, it is also not the case that the environment and behaviors are all to blame. Most people with lung cancer are or were smokers. But although smoking is one of the most health-damaging and dangerous behaviors one can do, most smokers do not get lung cancer; their genes protect them.

One of the most informative studies of the role of genes in stress and health comes from a group of approximately a thousand people born in Dunedin, New Zealand. These children were followed for about thirty years. Many developed depression but most did not.[95]

Some participants had genes that inclined them to have low levels of serotonin—the brain chemical that is boosted by antidepressant drugs like Prozac. Some individuals faced a number of stressful life events.

It turned out that risk of depression was predicted by a combination (or interaction) of a certain gene pattern and stressful challenges in life. If you had the risky genes but were on a healthy pathway, you didn't develop depression. If you faced stress but did not have the risky genes that increased your vulnerability, you again were unlikely to develop depression.

A similar situation is likely for many health risks involving stress. We have found not only that some people are more likely to encounter stress, but also that some are more likely to suffer detrimental consequences of the stress. What is special about the lifelong Terman study is that it reveals how one risk can lead to another and how patterns produce cumulative results.

The Fit with Other Veterans Studies

Our findings about the detrimental long-term effects of combat have been confirmed by other studies. The most analogous research project is Dr. George Vaillant's study of the lives of Harvard College men, which began in 1937 when they were sophomores. More than three-quarters of these men served in World War II. Like the Terman men, they varied quite a bit in how much combat they saw. Vaillant found that the men who faced intense hostilities were much more likely to face chronic diseases later. And like the Terman men and women, these traumatized veterans were much more likely to die at a younger age. Finally, Vaillant found that those who were the most stressed out in war were the most likely to develop symptoms of post-traumatic stress.[96]

A comparable study looked at several thousand American men who were army veterans from the Vietnam War era (1965–71). These veterans were interviewed and assessed in the 1980s and then followed for more than fifteen years.[97] Some had served at least one tour of duty in Vietnam, others had served elsewhere overseas, and still others had served only in the United States. This study, too, found that service in the war zone (Vietnam) raised the risk of postwar early mortality.

But other interesting confirmations appeared as well in the Vietnam veterans study. Those veterans who were not married, drank a lot, smoked, had lower incomes, and generally fit the pattern of someone heading off the healthy path were at higher risk. This was especially true if they suffered post-traumatic stress and were depressed. They were at higher risk not only of dying but also of dying in particular from cardiovascular disease. These American veterans of the war in Vietnam obviously grew up in a different time and faced different challenges than veterans of the Second World War. Yet the pathways to long life were pretty much the same. In fact, even a study of traumatic war experiences of veterans of the American Civil War (1861–65) showed such long-term stress-related effects on health.[98]

What It Means for You: Guideposts to Health and Long Life

The National World War II Memorial to American soldiers opened in Washington, D.C., in 2004, almost sixty years after the end of the war. Since its opening, many thousands of the veterans have visited the memorial and many others have added their names to the memorial's online archives. These are veterans who often faced serious stress and yet lived well into their eighties, nineties, and hundreds. What can we learn from them?

Our studies of the Terman participants have shown that the psychological stress of war itself is not necessarily a major health threat. Rather, it is the cascade of unhealthy patterns that sometimes follows. The more severe the stress, the more kinds of adaptation and coping are needed. Those soldiers isolated in far-off lands, seeing the most horrifying of combat scenarios, are at the most risk—and much the worse if they were already prone to unhealthy decisions and traveling a lonely, unhealthy pathway. The drinking, smoking, overeating, sleep disturbances, moodiness, and other signs of chronic stress often appear together and reinforce each other.

However, those individuals who can find meaning in a traumatic experience—such as going to war or facing a terrorist attack—and are able to reestablish a sense of security about the world are usually the ones who return to a healthy pathway.[99] Often this involves working with friends or colleagues to help make things better for others. For example, John teamed with his wartime friends to help provide scholarships to young veterans. On the behavioral side, those who did better were the ones who avoided drowning their sorrows and instead turned to sports, social clubs, and productive hard work.

The very most successful persons, however, are not those who simply react productively in *response* to stress, but those who put themselves on a better path from the get-go. Those individuals, as John and many of the other long-lived Terman participants demonstrated, are less likely to find themselves in stressful situations in the first place. And if they do encounter traumatic challenges, they are less likely to let the ensuing pressures take control of them; they use their existing tried-and-true means for heading off stress before it can become chronic and debilitating. They are motivated, persistent, and prudent. They take care of themselves, avoiding catastrophizing thoughts and working hard at life's challenges—even picking the weevils out of their cereal. And most important, they turn to the good social relationships that are the hallmark of their healthy life pathways.

CHAPTER 15

Individual Paths to Health and Long Life

(and Why We Won't Take Polypills)

A while back, we were contacted by the now-adult daughter of a long-lived Terman participant. She wanted to tell us how proud her father was to have been in this unique lifelong study, from the time he was first pulled out of his San Francisco classroom by Dr. Terman in 1921, and for all of his ninety-plus years. This conversation reminded us that we health researchers should not get so caught up in the fascinating findings that we forget about the bigger picture of why we are doing this work in the first place. After all, why conduct so much research on the longevity project unless we can draw some concrete conclusions about ways to improve individual health and longevity?[100]

Polypills: The Joke's on Us

Back when the new scientific field of health psychology was just getting formally organized as a modern science, those of us interested in this new research used to tell a running joke. It was about polypills. It was clear to us that health was being "overmedicalized." That is, every human ill, vice, and failing was being turned into a *disease* to be treated by doctors, usually with pills. And, in turn, it seemed almost every problem was giving rise to its own government agency. There is

the National Cancer Institute, the National Institute on Alcohol Abuse
and Alcoholism, the National Institute of Mental Health, the National
Institute on Drug Abuse, the National Institute on Deafness and
Other Communication Disorders, the National Center on Minority
Health and Health Disparities, and the National Institute on Aging
(which funded a lot of our own research).[101] There are many, many
others. Of course, these are all significant issues, very deserving of
scientific study. But don't they differ on many dimensions that should
be distinguished, and don't they overlap in many ways that should be
consolidated? That is, these National Institutes of Health are tremendously productive and well-run organizations, but are such divisions
the best way to address health, broadly understood?

The focus on specific diseases and treatments (in medical schools
and at the National Institutes of Health) is so strong that a new term
had to be invented to deal with health promotion and disease prevention. The word *wellness*—only several decades old—was invented,
broadcast, and popularized by humanists and social scientists to
counter the dehumanizing overuse of medical technology and the
overspecialization of physicians. Specialists could treat your disease,
but if you wanted to stay healthy or be treated as a whole person, you
would need to seek a promoter of wellness.

Many programs thus have been set up to promote *wellness.* But if
you think about it, what's wrong with the perfectly good word *health*?
What was wrong was that approaches to health were so tied up with
disease that scientists interested in the positive aspects of health had
to get away from the term and say they were studying wellness.

This confusion of health and disease led to many problems. People
began turning to physicians to deal with all sorts of difficulties that
traditionally had been addressed by friends, family elders, clergy members, chefs, coaches, hygienists, and mentors. Medical tests and procedures were sometimes applied to people who were basically fine, or
who needed some coaching, or who would get better with time and
healthy friendships. Many times physicians could help, but there were
also side effects, medical errors, and spiraling costs. Medical treat-

ment began consuming an ever-larger share of the gross domestic product. We could see that this would be impossible to maintain, and someday the sheer economic pressures would cause a reevaluation of this narrow view of health—that our day would come.

Health care became so focused on treating every problem with medication that we used to joke that someday someone would propose a huge pill full of potent medications, for everyone to take daily. Just think, with enough pharmaceutical collaboration, we could swallow one huge capsule each evening and treat cholesterol, overeating, alcoholism, insomnia, headaches, aging, depression, shyness, sunburn, hypertension, inattention, inactivity, and erectile dysfunction, all at once!

Distressingly enough, it now turns out that the joke was on us. There are real "polypills" under development and real proposals in circulation for "polypills" for everyone. Give all the world this huge pill and disease rates will plummet!

But not for us, because we know that there are often things you can do to configure your individual pathway to health and long life and to nudge yourself onto a smoother track. Targeted pills have helped millions and saved many lives; they are needed if you've developed a specific disease or condition that is clearly a threat to your life. But polypills—or any all-in-one quick fix—are a poor way to set most people on paths to long life.

There is no doubt that an unfortunate individual can be suddenly struck by a bus or by a virulent infection. There is no point in blaming the victim, and there is no way to have near-perfect control over your health. Many times, awful things happen for no rational reason. But, as we have discovered over and over in our studies, some pathways are much healthier than others, and many people have made their own luck by following them.

Most research on long life looks for the genes and the drugs that will delay aging. It is fascinating and important research but has no wonder pill for us. Ironically, many people overlook or misunderstand the less exotic but much more effective tools already at our disposal.

Secrets of the Body

The patterns and pathways to long life that we have uncovered make a significant difference in health and longevity—on average, many account for five or more years of life. If you put them together, you find the reasons why many bright, healthy children live to their seventies, eighties, and even nineties or hundreds, while many other bright, healthy children go on to die in their fifties and sixties.

It may be surprising to realize that there are only a few things that are reliably known to be directly and consistently bad for health. The complexities surrounding good health are the key reason why many touted remedies sound plausible but are merely folklore. What are the simple, direct threats, and what are the more subtle, complex ones?

The first direct threats are toxins (or poisons) in sufficient amounts. Inhaling cigarette (tobacco) smoke brings a toxic stew of chemicals into direct contact with sensitive internal organs. Ingesting lead (from lead paint or pollutants) or other heavy metals, or pesticides, or polluted air, clearly kills human cells and damages organs.

The second sort of direct threat to health is radioactivity. Too much exposure to radiation will make you sick or kill you, whether it is from radon in your basement, fallout from nuclear weapons or nuclear waste, or too many medical X-rays (especially CT scans) in your hospital. Radioactive exposure is cumulative, meaning that risk rises with each exposure.

The third kind of health threat is virulent infectious diseases—certain viruses, bacterial infections, and fungus infections—which start to overwhelm the body's natural defenses, especially when it's already weakened. Here is where health care resources are concentrated. That is, here is where our health system does a very good job of developing and providing vaccines, and where physicians do an excellent job of administering pharmaceutical treatments to fight serious infections.

The most obvious direct threats to health involve trauma—the car crashes that crush skulls, the drownings that suffocate lungs, and the gunshots that sever arteries. Here is where surgeons and emergency physicians provide modern medical miracles.

But then things start to get complicated. Significant genetic abnormalities, sometimes inherited and sometimes due to damage from the environment, cause an important amount of disease and death. But many times, the problem will only appear if the environmental circumstances allow or elicit it. For example, if you are genetically prone to certain allergies or to certain addictions or to depression, you have no problem if the allergen or the addictive substance or the triggering stress is not available to you.

When other common areas of health promotion enter the picture, everything is open for dispute—which foods to eat, which medications to take, how to limit stress, which screenings to ask for, which physical activities to engage in, and which personality traits will put you at risk. They are very relevant but not simple to sort out. Why is there so much uncertainty when it comes to these aspects of health?

The human body is in a constant state of change and development, and so any single intervention can have varying results. At the extremes, the effects are clear—not only is dehydration a problem but even drinking too much water can kill you. High stress is a problem but so is awful boredom. The correct balance is hard to know at a single point in time. This is why pathways—long life paths—are so important. The healthy Terman participants did not know much about exercise classes, meditation breaks, or happiness courses, even though exercise, stress, and mental health are important. Their healthy life pathways helped them stay on track, and when challenges knocked them off the route, they persisted in finding the way back.

Staying Healthy, Living Long: The Paths to Long Life

What have we learned about how to stay healthy and what individuals can do? First, take a deep breath. Second, take a deeper perspective.

The lives of the Terman participants revealed that it is not enough to focus on our bodies. Although individual bodies become ill, and doctors treat patients and not the friends and families of the patients, it is equally important to focus on families, work, and social relations. Social settings and social ties emerged as crucial components of health across the decades. Social relations deeply affect one's habits, daily activities, long-term plans, and reactions to challenges. The family environment, the divorce of one's parents, and the stresses of starting school too early all influenced the Terman children's health for years to come; and their health in old age was clearly linked to satisfaction with their careers, social networks, marital status, and friendships.

From a sophisticated scientific point of view, it makes no sense to think of a human body merely as an engine that needs to be oiled and tuned or as a plant that needs to be watered and fed. At its essence, individual health depends on social health.

Which Path?

One practical way to understand the threats to health and the likely best changes to be made is to match one's own inclinations to one of the paths we have discovered. The self-assessments provided in the previous chapters are helpful in generating a profile. Fill out the scales, gather up the scores, and create a view of the key contours of your life. There are many variations of healthy and unhealthy pathways, but here are some of the most common ones.

The High Road

If you are like Patricia, the conscientious sort with good friends and a happy marriage, you are likely on a very healthy pathway. The thoughtful planning and perseverance that such people invest in their relationships promote long life—naturally and automatically, even when challenges arise. Ironically, such prudent, persistent achievers with stable families and social support are usually the ones most concerned with what they should be doing to stay healthy. But they are already doing it.

We did not find that precisely living out your dreams matters much for your health. And being perfectly suited to one's job did not always predict a longer life. Instead it was again the thoughtful planning, sense of control and accomplishment, and perseverance that helped, often as encouraged by one's career successes.

Not Easy Street

Norris Bradbury, the scientist and Terman participant who oversaw the nation's nuclear arsenal for many years at a time of severe Cold War tension, was not enfeebled by the relentless strain he encountered. Yes, such individuals face adrenaline surges and high-pressure deadlines, but our studies found hard work and accomplishment to be a strong predictor of long life. Along with his wife of sixty-four years, children, grandchildren, and great-grandchildren, Bradbury thrived. Shelley Smith Mydans, the *Life* reporter, was a world traveler, prisoner of war, and often-threatened correspondent, yet she was not done in by stress. Those who were the most successful were the ones least likely to die at any given age. Ambition was not a problem and taking it easy was not healthy. In fact, those men who were carefree, undependable, and unambitious in childhood and very unsuccessful in their careers had a whopping increase in their mortality risk. On the other hand, if you have lots of responsibilities on the job but few resources and little cooperation from your coworkers, it is time for a change.

Off the Beaten Path

If you are like John, the shy scientist, then you may have found a lesser-known but still viable path to long life. Although he never married, John found much satisfaction and reward in his work. He had a small but stable group of friends with whom he maintained close contacts, and his career path complemented his personal strengths—attention to detail, persistence, and a love of learning. John, a truthful, sensitive, and shy boy, discovered his path to health through his scientific career. He kept in touch with his wartime buddies (from his stint in intelligence work) but mostly found his friends through his job. He was generous in helping and mentoring his colleagues and students, and he stayed healthy.

If you live near a technological research company, university, or think tank—the kind of place where John worked—here is an interesting experiment to understand better why John stayed healthy. First, look at the non-research-affiliated people in the surrounding community—how much they weigh, what they eat, how they behave, and so on. Then go into the research setting and observe the researchers. You will probably find that there is a huge difference between these engaged scientists and the intelligent people in the general public—a difference reflected in terms of obesity, drinking, smoking, social activities, and more. The resulting health differences are not due to any single cause, but to the overall psychosocial milieu. The scientists like John have a whole array of influences that bring them to and keep them on the healthy paths. A similar comparison could be made by observing a group of clergy. Or take a look at people who work on an organic farm or in a health club. The groups you associate with often determine the type of person you become. For people who want improved health, association with other healthy people is usually the strongest and most direct path of change.

James was not a scientist like John, but he found an analogous, if unorthodox, path to long life. Tactful and sociable but initially not very conscientious, James nevertheless was able to develop a maturity that increased each year. Although his parents divorced, he himself had a good marriage, completed his education, and stayed in touch with his sensitive side—by gradually developing a deep satisfaction and pride in his work and his hobbies, especially his music and stage work. Individuals with an artistic or philosophical bent stayed healthy if they continued to be physically active, steadily matured, and then remained responsible.

Catastrophe Lane

When someone like Dr. Douglas Kelley follows the example of his subject—the notorious Nazi Hermann Goering—and swallows cyanide, it is rarely a bolt out of the blue. For most suicides and other deaths due to violent recklessness, there are precursors and warning signs—available signals of dangerous pathways. Those in a mental downward spiral following a disappointment often forge a path characterized by drinking, anxiety, depression, and catastrophizing, with premonitions of accidents or violence. Although some may try to hide it with an unnatural joviality, those who fit this pattern can often be recognized; as with cheery Paul, they are either avoiding something troubling or are much too careless and carefree.

Heading down an unhealthy path shouldn't discourage anyone from attempting to bounce back. Those Terman participants who successfully took charge of their thoughts and stopped catastrophic thinking often returned to a more viable way, usually with the help of a spouse, therapist, or close friend.

Happy Trails to You

To an outsider, Paul—cheerful and sociable, masculine and well liked—seemed to have it all, but he lived an unfortunately foreshortened life. In contrast, Jess Oppenheimer had a difficult childhood—often picked on and fighting with schoolmates—but the ironic striving that resulted from his challenges served him well once he became a highly successful Hollywood comedy writer. He got married, became a father, and led a stable but very active and creative long life. One key difference between the two lay in the function of the jokester role. Jess learned to use humor in a warmhearted, meaningful way, showing human foibles but also the importance of relationships. For him it was also a tool with which to make a good living. For Paul, in contrast, it seems to have served a different function—one more selfish and sardonic. His optimistic, carefree attitude encouraged him to underestimate risks to his health and to approach his career goals in a lackadaisical fashion. It even hindered the sorts of close, social bonds that are so important to long life. He was the life of the party, but with few true confidants. We're not suggesting dampening your cheerfulness or humor, but rather challenging the idea that humor automatically causes health. In fact, as we saw, happiness does not cause good health; both happiness and health result from being on the right paths.

The Road Less Traveled

A striking theme emerged from our findings about those individuals—usually women—who often ignored social convention. Emma followed a life path that many young women of her era tried to avoid: She never married. She pursued her career with passion and her life was rewarding and full. She traveled. She was independent yet had a group of close friends (and her siblings) to share her joys and to encourage her during difficult times. Emma's reports to Terman over the years don't reflect a woman who felt her life was incomplete. Instead they suggest a spirited woman, very agreeable but serious, taking advantage of the opportunities afforded her. Although a good marriage can contribute to health and well-being, marriage can also bring troubles, plus the possibility of breakup and its health-damaging consequences.

Barbara, altruistic and agreeable, began her adulthood more conventionally than did Emma—she got married. But then she, too, headed down a less-traveled road. She was divorced, and she chose not to remarry. Like many of the women, but not the men, who divorced, she stayed healthy. She had close friends, as did Emma, and Barbara's career in social work provided her with many opportunities to reach out to others. As was the case for many of the Terman women, Barbara's life revealed an unexpected but common, healthy path for a woman—staying single after a divorce.

The Road to Resilience

The highly successful Hollywood director Edward Dmytryk, one of the hardest-working Terman subjects, led one of the most stressful lives yet lived to age ninety. Those who cared about others—who were agreeable but not necessarily sociable—often thrived even in the face of adversity. Like Dmytryk, they sought out the best in others, which was a key road to resilience. The same could be said of those children who faced the divorce of their parents. Those who got back on track, with a sense of accomplishment in their careers and a happy marriage of their own, lived long lives.

We didn't find that competition and drive are unhealthy characteristics. On the contrary, those who were the most disappointed with their achievements died the youngest. It would be naïve to think that successful Hollywood directors like Dmytryk, TV writers like Jess Oppenheimer, and the like cannot compete and throw an elbow at their opponent if needed. But they had the persistence, the motivation, and especially the support of a spouse or a close friend to come back each time they faced a challenge. Resilience was not a trait they were born with, nor an inner insight, but a process of perseverance and hard work.

The Long and Winding Road

Many of the Terman children were on a very healthy trajectory in the first third of their lives—they were more physically active (especially the boys), were well-adjusted, and had many friends and teammates. But by age sixty, most of them had lost vigor and energy (and tended now to resemble those who had been less active). Their childhood activity levels didn't translate directly to living longer. Instead, it was those who started active and stayed active, and those who started out less active but increased (and maintained) their activity, who lived the longest.

Staying physically active was clearly important to good health and long life. But it was not those who made resolutions to go running who succeeded. Rather, it was those whose habits, routines, and social networks encouraged movement and made it difficult to sit in one place who did well. The Terman participants lived most of their lives before the popular availability of jogging trails and marathons, gyms and treadmills, and running shoes and sweat-wicking athletic attire. Yet many stayed active, trim, and fit. Modern developments in the exercise industry can help individuals optimize and improve their fitness, but it is the broader patterns that lead one to maintain this fitness throughout many years.

An analogous finding emerged with conscientiousness. It was those who were conscientious as children and who remained highly persistent and prudent as adults who lived the longest. Nevertheless, those who started out unconscientious but entered positions requiring maturity and growth, and who increased their levels of prudence and persistence, were able to close much of the gap. Such patterns, common among the Terman subjects, revealed that there were inclinations and patterns launched in childhood, but little was fixed and determined at an early age. Rather, it was those who stayed on the healthiest paths, plus those who found their ways to the healthiest paths, who thrived in the second half of life.

The Feminine Avenue—Establishing Social and Emotional Ties

Many of the Terman men tended to rely on their wives for their social ties and their emotional health. When these were lost due to divorce or death, the consequences were often devastating. Among men, those who were in stable married relationships lived the longest. But the same was not true for the women. As noted, the women could more easily establish social and emotional ties with others. Those Terman subjects— male or female—who could nurture the feminine quality of social connectedness stayed healthier. The more masculine men *and* the more masculine women died sooner, while the more feminine women *and* the more feminine men lived longer.

The Less Sunny Side of the Street

Unlike catastrophizing, moderate worrying often conferred real benefits to health. James, tactful and sensitive, was something of a worrier throughout his life. But it turned out that his concerns prompted him to take better care of his health, especially after the death of his wife. Particularly for those with no spouse or close family member to urge them in the right direction, and especially for men, neurotic tendencies can promote longevity. Neurotic worrying as part of a syndrome of catastrophizing, anger, and depression was a sign of heightened risk, but for many people, nagging thoughts and irksome concerns were important to heading toward better health. This, too, was an unexpected finding that goes against common wisdom.

So there's no need for worriers to fret that this trait will threaten their health. Unless your worrying is disrupting your friendships or impairing your work, it can come in handy (and be health promoting) when you're facing various challenges needing thoughtful consideration.

The Holy Way

Religious individuals tend to live longer. In part, this is due to their healthier lifestyles, which is not at all surprising. And sometimes this long-life advantage is a phony finding, which emerges because some unhealthy people may be less able to be active in religious life. But what is it about religious involvement, especially for women, that goes beyond these simple matters? Feeling special and appreciated was not a key element of health. The calming aspects of prayer, meditation, and so on likewise did not emerge as of central importance, although they certainly help some individuals deal with acute stress. Instead it was that many religious individuals (and many nonreligious Terman subjects) were actively involved in their communities. They had close friends and social ties they could rely on. Those who were engaged with others lived longer lives.

Donna's life eventually followed the unholy way. Somewhat involved in religion during the first part of her life, she drifted away from her church over time. She was divorced, and busy with a demanding job in advertising, without much time for friends. This was congruent with her other more masculine characteristics. When she left her congregation, she created a real deficit in her life. People like Donna likely would have done much better if they had maintained close social contacts, whether through church organizations or similar groups. The divorce of her parents seems to have set her down a path in which one health threat followed another. Even a polypill would not have saved her.

The Persistent, Consequential, and Social Life

The 1,528 Terman participants were all quite intelligent, with a good start in life. By age ten they were doing well in school, were noticed by their teachers, and were being investigated by a Stanford professor—Lewis Terman. Many went on to be successful, but quite a large number of their fellow participants faced regular disappointments—in love, in careers, and in length of life. Some who succeeded were lucky, but many others made their own luck.

Across the life span, many predictors emerged as to who would do better and who would do worse, who would live longer and who would die younger. It was not good cheer or being popular and outgoing that made the difference. It was also not those who took life easy, played it safe, or avoided stress who lived the longest. Rather, it was those who—through an often-complex pattern of persistence, prudence, hard work, and close involvement with friends and communities—headed down meaningful, interesting life paths and, as we have illustrated, found their way back to these healthy paths each time they were pushed off the road.

The qualities and lifestyles cultivated by people on these long-life paths reflect an active pursuit of goals, a deep satisfaction with life, and a strong sense of accomplishment. That's not to say that these people possessed a giddy sense of happiness—we described how cheerfulness doesn't necessarily lead to a long life. But having a large social network, engaging in physical activities that naturally draw you in, giving back to your community, enjoying and thriving in your career, and nurturing a healthy marriage or close friendships can do more than add many years to your life. Together, they represent the living with purpose that comes from working hard, reaching out to others, and bouncing back from difficult times.

How fascinating to understand that those individuals who became involved with others in a consequential life would be improving their health as an unanticipated bonus. Of course many consequential lives have been cut tragically short, and some long lives seem bereft of accomplishment. Still, because getting and staying on healthy life paths can be a lifelong challenge, it is heartening to know that embracing the lessons of the Terman participants and striving for a socially richer and more productive life will increase the odds of a *long* life as well.

Long Life and Public Health

Looking Ahead to What Society Should Do

O ur research findings point to the startling conclusion that many
of the most cherished recommendations and policies about health
are misguided. This eight-decade study of the successful paths to
health and long life suggests that traditional approaches to health care
and health promotion have some disquieting deficiencies.

Health care costs are exploding while overall quality of health is
static. Many scientists predict that, for the first time, expected longevity will begin decreasing. They point to the failure of individuals to
follow medical advice to exercise, lose weight, sleep enough, wear sun-
screen, take it easy, eat right, be properly scanned, avoid illegal drugs,
and take enough prescribed pills on the proper schedules. We, however, are more optimistic. After spending two decades studying the
lives of the Terman participants, we see ways to turn things around.

Our findings about long life are now being tested, bit by bit, by
other researchers using different people—those born in later years, in
different subcultures, and in diverse populations. Yet the pathways to
long life seem very much the same. The most recent evidence suggests
that the core findings from the Terman studies are very relevant to
health today.

Lewis Terman died in 1956, just before his eightieth birthday. This
was quite a long life for someone of his generation, especially for
someone who had spent much of his early life suffering from recurring

tuberculosis (which eventually hastened his demise). Probably not co-incidentally, his wife had died earlier that same year, after more than fifty years of marriage. To the very end, he immensely enjoyed his contact with his subjects and remained in touch with almost all of them. A conscientious, active, and hardworking man who faced many stresses, Dr. Terman had set out to study the characteristics and successes of talented individuals, but he came to recognize that talent was much more complicated than he had imagined. The same might now be said about our understanding of the bases of health and longevity.

Wrong Ideas About Health

Policy makers and laypersons alike tend to make two major conceptual errors when thinking about health and longevity. First, people tend to overestimate the importance of family biology. Your height is heavily influenced by the genes you inherit from your parents, and your eye color is determined, but predicting your own health and longevity from that of your parents is mediocre at best. Sure, tendencies toward certain diseases run in families, and some diseases have clear genetic causes. This knowledge is helpful in choosing screening tests and having an idea which warning signs to watch for. But as a predictor of whether you will have a heart attack or live a long life? The experience of your relatives is not very precise at all. Your own life path matters more.

The second core error about health, which we've described in our research above, is the idea that we can make a major difference in health and longevity by giving people lists of health recommendations. We often hear physicians say, "Of course eat right, stop smoking, lose weight, sleep more, exercise, etc., etc., etc., should be the first choice in staying healthy but most of my patients can't do this, so it is a great thing that we have these effective medications." Such sentiments are perfectly natural, because if you hand most patients a list of life-altering changes, they will not make them.

The Terman participants who led long lives were never handed such a list. Yet they found their ways to healthy pathways. When a society's approach to health is dominated by threats and diseases, it pushes us to focus on things going wrong inside the individual's body—that is, on the infections, blockages, genetic aberrations, and hormonal and chemical imbalances. Our doctors then try to repair the problem. As we have repeatedly noted, for an acutely ill person, or for someone in deteriorating health, this approach can often work wonders—therein are the miracles of modern medicine. However, this approach is only part of the story, and the roads to long life are ignored at our peril.

Using data derived from the more than eighty years of the Terman study, and collecting and creating new information about the participants' lives, health, longevity, and causes of death, we have discovered many things we did not expect. We came to see the sometimes-complex but nonrandom pathways that link personalities, predispositions, behaviors, social groups, work environments, and health and longevity.

In contrast to finding a penicillin for infection or a clot-buster for stroke, simple "cures" for unconscientious personalities, marital instability, exposure to traumatizing stress, social isolation, workplace failures, and social-psychological anomie and estrangement are unlikely to be found in the clinic. Indeed, because individuals and their social groups change over time, the challenges likewise evolve.

Why Lists Don't Work So Well

When John Kennedy became president he immediately began emphasizing the importance of physical health and the role of government in promoting fitness. Fifty-mile hikes became a fad. This was the same year that Terman participant Dr. Ancel Keys, featured on the cover of *Time* magazine, told Americans that they ate too much. Now, half a century later, most segments of the American population are not only more obese but are less fit than ever. This doesn't mean that President

Kennedy's efforts were misguided or caused today's problems. But it does suggest that such traditional approaches are often ineffective over the long term.

Oversimplified recommendations may have made things worse. A while back, fear of fat emerged, as various well-meaning experts proclaimed the consumption of fat to be the big health hobgoblin. All sorts of low-fat foods were produced and marketed. Many people increased their carbohydrate intake instead. But fat and carbohydrate metabolism in the body is complicated, and it is not at all clear that a high-carbohydrate diet is healthy as a replacement. We are not sure of all the causes, but during the years since the health advisers began preaching against eating too much fat, the levels of obesity among Americans have increased dramatically.

Many other examples could be given of where "do this" or "don't do that" recommendations are overly simple checklists that later turn out to be too narrow, misleading, or deadly wrong. Even when the recommendations are well-founded, lists of recommendations often fail to have their intended effect. If you make a typical list of New Year's resolutions and head out on your own, you are highly unlikely to keep them over the long term.

Dr. Terman's Biases

When Lewis Terman began planning his major study back in 1919, American women could not vote, had limited property rights, and were excluded from many colleges. Most men and most women did not believe that women were or could be intellectual leaders equal to men, and neither did Terman. Yet to his credit, Terman included girls in his study.

African Americans, Latinos, Asian Americans, and others were often segregated into separate but unequal schools during this era, and likewise faced limited opportunities for college and advanced study. Dr. Terman made few if any efforts to find and include segregated minority groups in his studies. He was by no means a liberal-minded scholar, except in one key respect: He was enamored of data and he generally did not let his preconceptions bias the information on the 1,528 participants. He was careful in his data analyses. He documented both successes and failures. As times changed and his studies revealed certain conclusions, Terman changed his views. Although some scientists set out to use intelligence tests and achievement outcomes simply to further their preconceived political views, Dr. Terman generally presented loads and loads of facts.

The Mental-Physical Health Connection

Most societies allocate certain budgets of money and resources to strengthen the social fabric, economic potential, and mental health of their citizens—programs for education, to prevent drug abuse, to help families, to provide parks, and to offer job training and other programs to lift people out of poverty. Different pots of money and resources are allocated to health care, to train doctors, build hospitals, research disease, and provide health insurance or access to care. The implicit view is that most individuals will naturally stay healthy, but if by chance they get sick, then well-trained physicians should be available to treat them.

Our many years of study of the Terman participants have led us to a different conclusion. Our studies suggest that a society with more conscientious and goal-oriented citizens, well integrated into their communities, is likely to be a society of health and long life. Of course, this will be especially helpful if the community also has clean and safe air, water, and food, and good schools and safe streets; but few appreciate the extent to which mental health is the close companion of physical health. And few fully grasp the importance of helping to develop the social patterns that let each individual find an appropriate way forward, step by step.

A parallel set of conclusions has been reached by neuroscientists studying stress early in life. For example, researchers at Rockefeller University argue that biological disruptions early in life set forces in motion that appear as disease decades later.[102] It is too soon to know for sure how much of the health risk becomes embedded early on in our biological systems and how much depends on the subsequent psychological and social processes that occur throughout life. But the implications are similar: well-adjusted children growing up in a socially stable society are much more likely to become healthy, long-living adults.

When in September 1921, the talented, conscientious young schoolgirl named Patricia was pulled out of her San Francisco classroom to be tested by Dr. Terman, neither she nor her teacher nor Lewis Terman knew much about what paths would enable her and some of her classmates to live in good health for more than nine decades. Dr. Terman rarely mentioned the word *longevity*, but in 1947, with the study near its halfway point, he wrote, "it is still too early to estimate accurately the ultimate contribution of the group to science, scholarship, literature, and social welfare, or its ultimate fertility, longevity, insanity rate, and divorce incidence."[103] It's not too early anymore. We hope the guideposts on the path to long life illuminated by the Terman subjects will inspire changes in our social and health care systems that will help us all travel healthier passages. Our own future work will focus on the development and implementation of such policies.

· ACKNOWLEDGMENTS ·

Any significant scientific project in the health field involves a large number of colleagues and assistants, and we are truly grateful to those who helped us in our efforts. The major scientific collaborators in our various research studies are listed below in the section entitled "Research Collaborators." In addition, the coauthors and grant support of our relevant scientific research papers are listed in the references in the endnotes. Many other talented graduate students, undergraduate students, and other faculty colleagues also played a valuable research role in many of our studies. Our twenty-year research project built directly upon the eight-decade study Lewis Terman launched—and all the many dozens of contributors deserve thanks but cannot be individually named here.

Regarding the preparation of this book, we greatly appreciate the editorial suggestions made by our friends and associates, including Carlin Flora, Jhoshua Friedman, Joel Haldeman, Dr. Karen Shaw, Dr. Miriam Schustack, Rebecca Shiffman, and Michael Tyler. Eli Friedman provided advanced computer expertise. We thank our professional colleagues and support staff at the University of California, Riverside, and La Sierra University, especially Michael Yonezawa for expert library assistance and Mrs. Dianne Fewkes for research administrative support.

Our literary agent, Barbara Lowenstein, devoted her formidable expertise to this project. Finally, we thank the people at Hudson Street Press, especially Caroline Sutton, who had a clear vision for the direction of this book, and Anna Sternoff, who was heroically devoted to editing the myriad findings and conclusions and getting all the details just right.

RESEARCH
· COLLABORATORS ·

The findings reported in this book are based on twenty years of investigation by our research team, as well as our refinement and supplementation of over eight decades of data on the Terman participants. The following collaborators played a significant role in one or more of the studies. The interpretations and conclusions in this book are our own and have not been checked or endorsed by our research collaborators. Relevant research papers are referenced in the endnotes. Any opinions or errors herein are ours and not the responsibility of any research collaborator.

Dr. Joan S. Tucker completed her Ph.D. at the University of California, Riverside, in 1993 and is currently a senior behavioral scientist at the Rand Corporation in Santa Monica, California. She is one of the world's leading authorities on social relations, behavior, and health. Joan's particular focus in our Terman studies has been the marital stability and social networks of the participants, although she has played a vital role in many aspects of the project.

Dr. Carol Tomlinson-Keasey, in discussions with Howard Friedman starting in 1989, helped hatch the idea of a "short project" (six months or a year was the original plan) to look at personality and longevity in the Terman sample. Carol was a collaborator on many of the early studies conducted in our laboratory. In 1999 she became the founding chancellor for the University of California, Merced, the tenth campus in the UC system. She died in 2009.

Dr. Joseph E. Schwartz is a professor in the Department of Psychiatry and Behavioral Science at the Stony Brook University Medical Center and at the Columbia University Medical Center. Well-known in the field of advanced methodology of health research, Joe spearheaded our first study of childhood sociodemographic predictors of mortality risk and, as our team's initial biostatistician, played a major role in guiding our analytic strategies. Joe was Howard Friedman's roommate in graduate school.

Dr. Michael H. Criqui collaborated for many years as our team's physician-epidemiologist and is a professor and division chief of Family and Preventive Medicine at the University of California, San Diego's School of Medicine. An award-winning researcher in the epidemiology and prevention of cardiovascular disease, one of Mike's roles on this project has been supervising the nosologist's coding of all the Terman participants' death certificates. As a collaborator from the beginning, he played a crucial part in guiding our thinking on health behaviors and causes of death.

Dr. Richard A. Lippa is well-known for his studies on gender-related individual differences (masculinity/femininity) and various personality, cognitive, and social dimensions. He is currently a professor of psychology at the California State University in Fullerton. Richard created the gender diagnosticity measures and collaborated with us as we uncovered the health risks associated with masculinity among the Terman participants.

Dr. Michael E. McCullough is a well-known expert on religion, forgiveness, and gratitude, currently at the University of Miami. Mike had the idea to examine the development and change in religious involvement among the Terman participants and then combine that information with our studies of their personalities, social ties, and longevity. He and his colleague Dr. Craig Enders brought their substantial expertise in the area of statistical modeling to bear on our study of the Terman participants' religious involvement over time.

Dr. Glen H. Elder, Jr., is a research professor of sociology and psychology at the University of North Carolina at Chapel Hill and an influential intellectual leader specializing in development over the life course. He was especially interested in the later-life outcomes of Terman participants who were part of the World War II effort and, along with his research team (Dr. James Scott Brown and the late Dr. Elizabeth Clipp), collaborated on our study on this topic.

Dr. Daniel R. Seldin completed his Ph.D. at the University of California, Riverside in 1999, and contributed especially to our analyses related to sexual activity and to careers. He now works in program evaluation.

Dr. Kathleen M. Clark completed her Ph.D. at the University of California, Riverside in 2000, and was a key researcher during the middle years of our twenty-year project, contributing to numerous studies. She is now a research director at a major health care company.

Dr. Keiko A. Taga completed her Ph.D. at the University of California, Riverside in 2006, and contributed significantly to our studies of bereavement and social support.

Dr. Margaret L. (Peggy) Kern in 2010 completed her Ph.D. at the University of California, Riverside. Peggy is a core collaborator on many important aspects of the research, including especially the physical activity studies, the work on early education, the work on career success, and the studies of healthy aging.

Dr. Chandra A. Reynolds is a psychology professor at the University of California, Riverside, and a leading expert on longitudinal statistical analyses and life-span developmental psychology. Chandra innovated and helped implement many of the data analyses involving change over time, as well as collaborating in important ways on studies of physical activity, careers, and partner effects.

Loryana Vie is a graduate student at the University of California, Riverside, who worked especially on the studies of marital happiness and health.

Other important collaborators include: **Dr. Deborah L. Wingard**, professor of Family and Preventive Medicine at the University of California, San Diego, an expert on epidemiology and women's health, who was a key contributor to a number of studies during the first five years of our project; **Dr. Catherine M. Tsai**, who worked on our study of playing with pets and longevity and then headed off to medical school; **Dr. Sharon Edelstein**, a biostatistician who helped with many of the initial life-span longevity analyses; **Dr. Charlotte N. Markey**, who completed her Ph.D. at the University of California, Riverside, and worked on several of our studies of life-span health; **Dr. Renee Goodwin**, an epidemiologist at Columbia University, who worked on the study of conscientiousness and chronic disease; **Dr. Christopher Peterson** of the University of Michigan and **Dr. Martin E. P. Seligman** of the University of Pennsylvania, who collaborated on our study of catastrophizing and are among the founders of the field of positive psychology; and **Gloria Luong**, who had the rare distinction of coauthoring a major scientific paper while still an undergraduate and who is now a graduate student in psychology.

In addition to our own research, we relied, of course, on the efforts of the late Dr. Lewis Terman and his many associates and successors. They are far too numerous to identify, but we would especially like to note the efforts of Mrs. Eleanor Walker, formerly of Stanford University, who assisted us with many of our initial forays into the original archives, and the many scholars associated with Dr. Terman or his project, especially including Melita Oden, Dr. Robert R. Sears, Dr. Al Hastorf, and Dr. Ed Shneidman.

· NOTES ·

Introduction

1. Lucille Ball's secret to staying young is quoted in A. Adams, *An Uncommon Scold* (New York: Simon and Schuster, 1989), 17. Regarding the matter of eating fast (among the Terman participants), relevant information was recorded during a comprehensive medical exam the children underwent in 1922 in either San Francisco or Los Angeles. About half the boys and more than a third of the girls were classified as fast eaters. When we analyzed the longevity data eighty-five years later, we found absolutely no indication that eating slowly promotes longevity.

2. The *New York Times* obituary of Shelley Smith Mydans was published on March 9, 2002.

Chapter 1: Personality and Long Life

3. In this book, we report our major findings in terms of group associations, common trajectories, and pathways to long life. When we present descriptions of Terman participants who have been publicly identified (such as Jess Oppenheimer and Shelley Smith Mydans), the information is factual and unaltered. When we use confidential case studies to illustrate key points, we use pseudonyms and alter some of the details in unimportant ways, so as not to breach the confidentiality that Terman promised the children and their parents. Dr. Terman used the same sorts of disguise when he presented anecdotes to illustrate his findings.

4. For a textbook on modern approaches to personality, see H. S. Friedman and M. W. Schustack, *Personality: Classic Theories and Modern Research*, 4th edition (Boston: Pearson Allyn and Bacon, 2009).

Chapter 2: Long Live the Prudent and Persistent

5. The self-assessments in this book are provided to help the reader gain a deeper understanding of the concepts under discussion. They are not intended or suitable for clinical or therapeutic use. Scoring is approximate.
6. The quote "Any fool can criticize . . ." comes from Dale Carnegie's 1936 book *How to Win Friends and Influence People*. It is often erroneously attributed to Benjamin Franklin.
7. For the details of our scale validation using modern measures, see for example L. R. Martin and H. S. Friedman, "Comparing Personality Scales across Time: An Illustrative Study of Validity and Consistency in Life-Span Archival Data," *Journal of Personality* 68 (2000): 85–110.
8. For our study of conscientiousness in childhood and adulthood, see L. R. Martin, H. S. Friedman, and J. E. Schwartz, "Personality and Mortality Risk across the Lifespan: The Importance of Conscientiousness as a Biopsychosocial Attribute," *Health Psychology* 26 (2007): 428–36.
9. For information on Yisroel Lipkin (Rav Yisroel Salanter), see D. Katz, *The Musar Movement: Its History, Leading Personalities and Doctrines* (Tel Aviv: Orly Press, 1975); or I. Salanter, I. Blaser, Z. Miller, and E. Linas, *Ohr Yisrael: The Classic Writings of Rav Yisrael Salanter and His Disciple Rav Yitzchak Blazer* (Southfield, MI: Targum, 2004).
10. For our scientific review of conscientiousness and long life, see M. L. Kern and H. S. Friedman, "Do Conscientious Individuals Live Longer? A Quantitative Review," *Health Psychology* 27 (2008): 505–12.
11. For our study with epidemiologist Renee Goodwin, see R. G. Goodwin and H. S. Friedman, "Health Status and the Five Factor Personality Traits in a Nationally Representative Sample," *Journal of Health Psychology* 11 (2006): 643–54.

Chapter 3: Friendly and Convivial

12. Details of our study on the longevity of scientists vs. nonscientists can be found in H. S. Friedman, J. S. Tucker, L. R. Martin, C. Tomlinson-Keasey, J. E. Schwartz, D. L. Wingard, and M. H. Criqui, "Do Non-scientists Really Live Longer?" *The Lancet* 343 (1994): 296.
13. We described our findings on personality and health behaviors in J. S. Tucker, H. S. Friedman, C. Tomlinson-Keasey, J. E. Schwartz, D. L. Wingard, M. H. Criqui, and L. R. Martin, "Childhood Psychosocial Predictors of Adulthood Smoking, Alcohol Consumption, and Physical Activity," *Journal of Applied Social Psychology* 25 (1995): 1884–99.

14. For more on personality and reward seeking, see Philip J. Corr, ed., *The Reinforcement Sensitivity Theory of Personality* (New York: Cambridge University Press, 2008). Also see C. Davis, K. Patte, R. Levitan, C. Reid, S. Tweed, and C. Curtis, "From Motivation to Behaviour: A Model of Reward Sensitivity, Overeating, and Food Preferences in the Risk Profile for Obesity," *Appetite* 48 (2007): 12–19.

Chapter 4: Happiness and Health?

15. For an article on psychotherapy and cancer, see J. C. Coyne, B. D. Thombs, M. Stefanek, S. C. Palmer, "Time to Let Go of the Illusion That Psychotherapy Extends the Survival of Cancer Patients: Reply to Kraemer, Kuchler, and Spiegel," *Psychological Bulletin* 135, no. 2 (2009): 179–82.

16. The J. D. Salinger quote is from *Raise High the Roof Beam, Carpenters and Seymour: An Introduction* (Boston: Little, Brown, 1959), 88.

17. For one of our studies of cheerfulness and longevity, see L. R. Martin, H. S. Friedman, J. S. Tucker, C. Tomlinson-Keasey, M. H. Criqui, and J. E. Schwartz, "A Life Course Perspective on Childhood Cheerfulness and Its Relation to Mortality Risk," *Personality and Social Psychology Bulletin* 28 (2002): 1155–65.

18. Anne Harrington provides a relevant history of mind-body matters in *The Cure Within: A History of Mind-Body Medicine* (New York: W. W. Norton, 2008).

19. The average person tends to rate his or her risk as below average. For further discussion of related matters, see N. D. Weinstein, "Exploring the Links between Risk Perceptions and Preventive Health Behavior," in *Social Psychological Foundations of Health and Illness*, ed. J. Suls and K. Wallston, 22–53 (Oxford, England: Blackwell, 2003).

20. For a study of aging and positive feelings, see M. Mather and L. Carstensen, "Aging and Motivated Cognition: The Positivity Effect in Attention and Memory," *Trends in Cognitive Sciences* 9 (2005): 496–502.

21. You can read more about Dr. Vaillant's study of the Harvard men in G. E. Vaillant, *Aging Well: Surprising Guideposts to a Happier Life from the Landmark Harvard Study of Adult Development* (Boston: Little, Brown, 2002).

22. For an overview of the Nun Study, see David Snowdon's *Aging with Grace: What the Nun Study Teaches Us about Leading Longer, Healthier, and More Meaningful Lives* (New York: Bantam, 2002).

23. For more information on the first study we mention on the protective effect of neuroticism, see A. E. Korten, A. F. Jorm, Z. Jiao, L. Letenneur, P. A. Jacomb, A. S. Henderson, H. Christensen, and B. Rodgers, "Health, Cognitive, and Psychosocial Factors as Predictors of Mortality in an Elderly Community Sample," *Journal of Epidemiology and Community Health* 53 (1999): 83–88. The second study, of (older) Medicare patients, is A. Weiss and P. T. Costa, Jr., "Domain and Facet Personality Predictors of All-Cause Mortality among Medicare Patients Aged 65 to 100," *Psychosomatic Medicine* 67 (2005): 724–33.
24. For a good relevant discussion of narcissism, see Jean M. Twenge, *Generation Me: Why Today's Young Americans Are More Confident, Assertive, Entitled—and More Miserable Than Ever Before* (New York: The Free Press, 2006).

Chapter 5: Catastrophic Thinking

25. To read more about our initial study of catastrophizing, see C. Peterson, M. E. P. Seligman, K. H. Yurko, L. R. Martin, and H. S. Friedman, "Catastrophizing and Untimely Death," *Psychological Science* 9 (1998): 127–30.
26. For more information on the risks associated with catastrophizing, see C. Peterson, S. F. Maier, and M. E. P. Seligman, *Learned Helplessness: A Theory for the Age of Personal Control* (New York: Oxford University Press, 1993).
27. For a brief biography of Dr. Douglas Kelley, see University of California: *In Memoriam*, 1959, "Douglas McGlashan Kelley, Criminology: Berkeley." See also "Mysterious Suicide of Nuremburg Psychiatrist," *San Francisco Chronicle*, p. A17, February 6, 2005. The *New York Times* article of January 2, 1958, is titled "U.S. Psychiatrist in Nazi Trial Dies," p. 18.
28. For Dr. Tomlinson-Keasey's study of these eight women see C. Tomlinson-Keasey, L. W. Warren, and J. E. Elliott, "Suicide among Gifted Women: A Prospective Study," *Journal of Abnormal Psychology* 95 (1986): 123–30.
29. To read more about Dr. Shneidman's investigation into the lives of these men who shot themselves, see E. Shneidman, "Perturbation and Lethality as Precursors of Suicide in a Gifted Group," *Life-Threatening Behavior* 1 (1971): 23–45. See also Shneidman's book *The Suicidal Mind* (New York: Oxford University Press, 1998).
30. The Cornell research on the regrets of the Terman participants is in N. Hattaiangadi, V. H. Medvec, and T. Gilovich, "Failing to Act: Regrets

of Terman's Geniuses," *International Journal of Aging and Human Development* 40 (1995): 175–85.

31. David Lester did a follow-up study on the Terman suicides, matched controls, and childhood personality; see D. Lester, "Completed Suicide in the Gifted," *Journal of Abnormal Psychology* 100 (1991): 604–6.

32. The study on adherence and health outcomes after heart attack is R. I. Horwitz, C. M. Viscoli, L. Berkman, R. M. Donaldson, S. M. Horwitz, C. J. Murray, D. F. Ransohoff, and J. Sindelar, "Treatment Adherence and Risk of Death after a Myocardial Infarction," *Lancet* 336, no. 8714 (1990): 542–45.

Chapter 6: Childhood and School Days

33. For our breast-feeding study see D. L. Wingard, K. H. Criqui, S. Edelstein, J. Tucker, C. Tomlinson-Keasey, J. E. Schwartz, and H. S. Friedman,"Is Breast-Feeding in Infancy associated with Adult Longevity?" *American Journal of Public Health* 84 (1994): 1458–62.

34. For our study of early education and long life, see: M. L. Kern and H. S. Friedman, "Early Educational Milestones as Predictors of Lifelong Academic Achievement, Midlife Adjustment, and Longevity," *Journal of Applied Developmental Psychology* 30 (2009): 419–30.

35. The Lee Cronbach details are from the "biographical memoirs" Richard J. Shavelson wrote up and published in the December 2003 *Proceedings of the American Philosophical Society* 147, no. 4.

Chapter 7: Parental Divorce

36. For the complete results of our first study showing that parental divorce predicted mortality risk years into the future see J. E. Schwartz, H. S. Friedman, J. S. Tucker, C. Tomlinson-Keasey, D. L. Wingard, and M. H. Criqui, "Sociodemographic and Psychosocial Factors in Childhood as Predictors of Adult Mortality," *American Journal of Public Health* 85, no. 9 (1995): 1237–45.

37. Our follow-up study, investigating the reasons why parental divorce is so important to later mortality risk, was published as J. S. Tucker, H. S. Friedman, J. E. Schwartz, M. H. Criqui, C. Tomlinson-Keasey, D. L. Wingard, and L. R. Martin, "Parental Divorce: Effects on Individual Behavior and Longevity," *Journal of Personality and Social Psychology* 73 (1997): 381–91.

38. For a study on parental divorce and cancer see K. Hemminki and B. Chen, "Lifestyle and Cancer: Effect of Parental Divorce," *European Journal of Cancer Prevention* 15, no. 6 (2006): 524–30.

39. For more about risky families see R. L. Repetti, S. E. Taylor, and T. E. Seeman, "Risky Families: Family Social Environment and the Mental and Physical Health of Offspring," *Psychological Bulletin* 128 (2002): 330–66.

40. You can read more about our findings on family environment and parental divorce in L. R. Martin, H. S. Friedman, K. M. Clark, and J. S. Tucker, "Longevity following the Experience of Parental Divorce," *Social Science and Medicine* 61 (2005): 2177–89.

41. For further research on effects of divorce over time see P. R. Amato, L. S. Loomis, and A. Booth, "Parental Divorce, Marital Conflict, and Offspring Well-Being during Early Adulthood," *Social Forces* 73 (1995), 895–915.

42. For more on possible genetic contributions to outcomes following parental divorce see B. M. D'Onofrio, E. Turkheimer, R. E. Emery, W. S. Slutske, A. C. Heath, P. A. Madden, and N. G. Martin, "A Genetically Informed Study of the Processes underlying the Association between Parental Marital Instability and Offspring Adjustment," *Developmental Psychology* 42, no. 3 (2006): 486–99.

Chapter 8: Running for Their Lives

43. For more on the K ration see Franz A. Koehler, "Special Rations for the Armed Forces, 1946–53," QMC Historical Studies, Series II, No. 6, Historical Branch, Office of the Quartermaster General, Washington, DC, 1958.

44. For one of our studies of physical activity, see M. L. Kern, C. A. Reynolds, and H. S. Friedman, "Predictors of Physical Activity Patterns across Adulthood: A Growth Curve Analysis," *Personality and Social Psychology Bulletin* (in press, 2010).

45. The Mark Twain quotes are at http://www.pbs.org/marktwain/learnmore/writings_seventieth.html.

46. Read more about patterns of physical activity over time in H. S. Friedman, L. R. Martin, J. S. Tucker, M. H. Criqui, M. L. Kern, and C. Reynolds, "Stability of Physical Activity across the Lifespan," *Journal of Health Psychology* 13 (2008): 966–78.

47. Neil Armstrong made this comment in an interview with news anchor Walter Cronkite, included in L. Eisenberg's *Fifty Who Made the Differ-*

ence: A Celebration of Fifty American Originals (New York: Random House, 1984).

48. To read more about METs and differences among groups, see M. A. Martinez-Gonzalez, J. A. Martinez, F. B. Hu, M. J. Gibney, and J. Kearney, "Physical Activity, Sedentary Lifestyle and Obesity in the European Union," *International Journal of Obesity and Related Metabolic Disorders* 23 (1999): 1192–1201.

49. For a study of the B vitamins, see C. M. Albert, N. R. Cook, J. M. Gaziano, E. Zaharris, J. MacFadyen, E. Danielson, J. E. Buring, and J. E. Manson, "Effect of Folic Acid and B Vitamins on Risk of Cardiovascular Events and Total Mortality among Women at High Risk for Cardiovascular Disease: A Randomized Trial," *Journal of the American Medical Association* 299, no. 17 (2008): 2027–36.

50. This study of aspirin and heart attack is H. D. Lewis, J. W. Davis, D. G. Archibald, W. E. Steinke, T. C. Smitherman, J. E. Doherty, H. W. Schnaper, M. LeWinter, E. Linares, J. M. Pouget, S. C. Sabharwal, E. Chesler, and H. DeMots, "Protective Effects of Aspirin against Acute Myocardial Infarction and Death in Men with Unstable Angina: Results of a Veterans Administration Cooperative Study," *New England Journal of Medicine* 309, no. 7 (1983): 396–403.

Chapter 9: To Sickness or to Health?

51. To read about Holmes and Rahe's original scale see T. H. Holmes and R. H. Rahe, "The Social Readjustment Rating Scale," *Journal of Psychosomatic Research* 11, no. 2 (1967): 213–18.

52. For further reading on our initial study of marital history and long life, see J. S. Tucker, H. S. Friedman, D. L. Wingard, and J. E. Schwartz, "Marital History at Midlife as a Predictor of Longevity: Alternative Explanations to the Protective Effect of Marriage," *Health Psychology* 15 (1996): 94–101.

53. From H. L. Mencken, *A Little Book in C Major* (New York: John Lane, 1916), 14.

54. For a discussion of marriage and happiness see R. E. Lucas and A. E. Clark, "Do People Really Adapt to Marriage?" *Journal of Happiness Studies* 7 (2006): 405–26.

55. The South Carolina study is described in D. A. Sbarra and P. J. Nietert, "Divorce and Death," *Psychological Science* 20 (2009): 107–13.

56. Our study of marital patterns is J. S. Tucker, J. E. Schwartz, K. M. Clark,

and H. S. Friedman, "Age-Related Changes in the Associations of Social Network Ties with Mortality Risk," *Psychology and Aging* 14, no. 4 (1999): 564–71.

57. Regarding marital happiness, see L. Vie, M. L. Kern, C. A. Reynolds, and H. S. Friedman, "Marital Happiness as a Predictor of Healthy Aging," presented Nov. 20, 2009 at the Annual Scientific Meeting of the Gerontological Society of America, Atlanta, Ga.

58. For an overview of studies on marriage and health, see J. K. Kiecolt-Glaser and T. L. Newton, "Marriage and Health: His and Hers," *Psychological Bulletin* 127, no. 4 (2001): 472–503.

59. Ibid.

60. The Terman "orgasm adequacy" phrase is from L. M. Terman and M. H. Oden, *Genetic Studies of Genius*, vol. 4, *The Gifted Child Grows Up: Twenty-five Years' Follow-up of a Superior Group* (Stanford, CA: Stanford University Press, 1947), 249.

61. Our study of sexual activity and long life is D. R. Seldin, H. S. Friedman, and L. R. Martin, "Sexual Activity as a Predictor of Life-Span Mortality Risk," *Personality and Individual Differences* 33 (2002): 409–25.

62. For other studies on sexual activity and health see G. D. Smith, S. Frankel, and J. Yarnell, "Sex and Death: Are They Related? Findings from the Caerphilly Cohort Study," *BMJ* 315 (1997): 1641–44; and H. K. Chen, C. D. Tseng, S. C. Wu, T. K. Lee, and T. H. H. Chen, "A Prospective Cohort Study on the Effect of Sexual Activity, Libido and Widowhood on Mortality among the Elderly People: 14-Year Follow-up of 2453 Elderly Taiwanese," *International Journal of Epidemiology* 36 (2007): 1136–42.

Chapter 10: Careers, Success, and Satisfaction

63. For an interesting article about Edward Dmytryk, see Richard English, "What Makes a Hollywood Communist?" *Saturday Evening Post*, May 19, 1951. For his *New York Times* obituary, see "Edward Dmytryk, Film Director, Dies at 90," July 3, 1999. His 1978 autobiography is *It's a Hell of a Life but Not a Bad Living* (New York Times Books).

64. For an overview of personality, immunity, and disease, see H. S. Friedman, "The Multiple Linkages of Personality and Disease," *Brain, Behavior, and Immunity* 22 (2008): 668–75. Also see M. E. Kemeny, "Psychoneuroimmunology," in *Foundations of Health Psychology*, ed. H. S. Friedman and R. C. Silver, 92–116 (New York: Oxford University Press, 2007).

65. The Terman quote is from Terman and Oden, *Genetic Studies of Genius*, vol. 4, *The Gifted Child Grows Up*, 314 (Stanford University Press, 1997).

66. The *New York Times* obituary for Norris Bradbury was published on August 22, 1997.

67. Peggy Kern, Chandra Reynolds, and Gloria Luong worked with us on this research. Gloria had the rare distinction of coauthoring our major scientific paper while still an undergraduate. For one of our papers on the longevity of the successful men, see M. L. Kern, H. S. Friedman, L. R. Martin, C. A. Reynolds, and G. Luong, "Conscientiousness, Career Success, and Longevity: A Lifespan Analysis," *Annals of Behavioral Medicine* 37 (2009): 154–63.

68. The study of career progression is E. K. Pavalko, G. H. Elder, and E. C. Clipp, *Journal of Health and Social Behavior* 34 (1993): 363–80.

69. Robert Sears, himself a Terman participant, had taken over certain responsibilities for the study and made major contributions to the database, including looking into this aspect of career satisfaction. See R. R. Sears, "Sources of Life Satisfactions of the Terman Gifted Men," *American Psychologist* 32 (1977): 119–28.

70. To read more about Melita Oden's life, see "Melita Oden, 95, Researcher, Caretaker of Saratoga's History" in the *San Jose Mercury News* (CA), April 21, 1993.

71. Terman's preface thanking Mrs. Oden is in Terman and Oden, *Genetic Studies of Genius*, vol. 4, *The Gifted Child Grows Up*, xi.

72. The report of picking the weevils is in *Time* magazine, December 31, 1945.

73. To read more about Dr. Holland's system of classification, see J. L. Holland, *The Psychology of Vocational Choice: A Theory of Personality Types and Model Environments* (Waltham, MA: Blaisdell, 1966).

74. For a study of personality, productivity, and longevity see H. S. Friedman, M. L. Kern, and C. A. Reynolds, "Personality and Health, Subjective Well-Being, and Longevity," *Journal of Personality* 78 (2010): 179–215.

75. The study of meaningful jobs and happiness is S. Lyubomirsky, L. A. King, and E. Diener, "The Benefits of Frequent Positive Affect: Does Happiness Lead to Success?" *Psychological Bulletin* 131 (2005): 803–55.

Chapter 11: Long Life Meets the Afterlife

76. For a review of religion and health see M. E. McCullough, W. T. Hoyt, D. B. Larson, H. G. Koenig, and C. E. Thoresen, "Religious Involvement and Mortality: A Meta-Analytic Review," *Health Psychology* 19 (2000): 211–22.

77. For philosopher David Hume's essay, see *An Enquiry concerning Human Understanding*, published in 1748.

78. Our study with Dr. McCullough is M. E. McCullough, H. S. Friedman, C. K. Enders, and L. R. Martin, "Does Devoutness Delay Death? Psychological Investment in Religion and Its Association with Longevity in the Terman Sample," *Journal of Personality and Social Psychology* 97 (2009): 866–82. For more reading on Dr. McCullough's work, see his book *Beyond Revenge: The Evolution of the Forgiveness Instinct* (San Francisco: Jossey-Bass, 2008).

79. For the large-scale, seven-year women's health study, see E. Schnall, S. Wassertheil-Smoller, C. Swencionis, V. Zemon, L. Tinker, M. J. O'Sullivan, L. Van Horn, and M. Goodwin, "The Relationship between Religion and Cardiovascular Outcomes and All-Cause Mortality in the Women's Health Initiative Observational Study," *Psychology and Health* 25, no. 2 (2010): 249–63.

Chapter 12: Confidants, Networks, and the Power of Social Life

80. Last year, in a funny episode, we were approached by a confused insect specialist from another university who wanted advice on how to set up a computer model for social networking based on the typical behaviors of those most social of insects, termites. We had to explain to him that we don't study the insect termites but the human ones—Terman's "Termites." But we were able to add that just as insect termites help ensure the survival of their colonies through cooperation and self-sacrifice, human "Termites" in social networks who lend a hand to others are helping to ensure their own survival.

81. The Defoe quote comes from *The Character of the Late Dr. Samuel Annesley, by Way of Elegy* (London: E. Whitlock, 1697).

82. We describe our study regarding pets in more detail in J. S. Tucker, H. S. Friedman, C. M. Tsai, and L. R. Martin, "Playing with Pets and Longevity among the Elderly," *Psychology and Aging* 10 (1995): 3–7.

Chapter 13: The Gender Gap in Long Life

83. Dr. Terman's explanation of the fact that scoring similarly to someone of the opposite sex was not diagnostic of homosexuality is in Terman and Oden, *Genetic Studies of Genius*, vol. 4, *The Gifted Child Grows Up*, 201.

84. For one of our studies of gender and longevity, see R. A. Lippa, L. R. Martin, and H. S. Friedman, "Gender-Related Individual Differences and Mortality in the Terman Longitudinal Study: Is Masculinity Hazardous to Your Health?" *Personality and Social Psychology Bulletin* 26 (2000): 1560–70.

85. For a discussion of social roles and mortality risk see I. Waldron, "Contributions of Changing Gender Differences in Behavior and Social Roles to Changing Gender Differences in Mortality," in *Men's Health and Illness: Gender, Power, and the Body*, ed. D. Sabo and D. F. Gordon, 22–45 (Thousand Oaks, CA: Sage, 1995).

86. Our initial report on the importance of stable moods for boys is in J. E. Schwartz, H. S. Friedman, J. S. Tucker, C. Tomlinson-Keasey, D. Wingard, and M. H. Criqui, "Sociodemographic and Psychosocial Factors in Childhood as Predictors of Adult Mortality," *American Journal of Public Health* 85 (1995): 1237–45.

87. For more information on the relationship between mental difficulties and mortality risk see L. R. Martin, H. S. Friedman, J. S. Tucker, J. E. Schwartz, M. H. Criqui, D. L. Wingard, and C. Tomlinson-Keasey, "An Archival Prospective Study of Mental Health and Longevity," *Health Psychology* 14 (1995): 381–87.

88. More on sex differences in health are in the following three articles: C. M. Gijsbers van Wijk, K. P. van Vliet, A. M. Kolk, and W. T. Everaerd, "Symptom Sensitivity and Sex Differences in Physical Morbidity: A Review of Health Surveys in the United States and the Netherlands," *Women and Health* 17 (1991): 91–124; L. M. Verbrugge, "The Twain Meet: Empirical Explanations of Sex Differences in Health and Mortality," *Journal of Health and Social Behavior* 30 (1989): 282–304; and K. S. Rook, S. T. Charles, and J. Heckhausen, "Aging and Health," in *Foundations of Health Psychology*, ed. H. S. Friedman and R. C. Silver, 234–62 (New York: Oxford University Press, 2007).

89. Other, shorter-term studies have also found that widowed women often live longer. See for example P. Lichtenstein, M. Gatz, and S. Berg, "A Twin Study of Mortality after Spousal Bereavement," *Psychological Medicine* 28 (1998): 635–43; and C. F. Mendes de Leon, S. V. Kasl, and S. Jacobs, "Widowhood and Mortality Risk in a Community Sample of the Elderly: A Prospective Study," *Journal of Clinical Epidemiology* 46 (1993): 519–27.

90. These dramatic findings about bereavement were first published in K. T. Taga, H. S. Friedman, and L. R. Martin, "Early Personality Traits as Pre-

dictors of Mortality Risk following Conjugal Bereavement," *Journal of Personality* 77 (2009): 669–90.

Chapter 14: The Toll of War and Trauma

91. For more about our core study on the Terman veterans, see G. H. Elder, E. C. Clipp, J. S. Brown, L. R. Martin, and H. S. Friedman, "The Life-Long Mortality Risks of World War II Experiences," *Research on Aging* 31 (2009): 391–412.

92. For discussions of the disease-prone personality, see H. S. Friedman and S. Booth-Kewley, "The 'Disease-Prone Personality': A Meta-Analytic View of the Construct," *American Psychologist* 42 (1987): 539–55; H. S. Friedman, "Personality, Disease, and Self-Healing," in *Foundations of Health Psychology*, ed. H. S. Friedman and R. C. Silver, 172–99 (New York: Oxford University Press, 2007); and H. S. Friedman, "The Multiple Linkages of Personality and Disease," *Brain, Behavior, and Immunity* 22 (2008): 668–75.

93. The large national study of depression in heart attack patients can be found at L. F. Berkman, J. Blumenthal, M. Burg, R. M. Carney, D. Catellier, M. J. Cowan, S. M. Czajkowski, R. DeBusk, J. Hosking, A. Jaffe, P. G. Kaufmann, P. Mitchell, J. Norman, L. H. Powell, J. M. Raczynski, and N. Schneiderman, "The Enhancing Recovery in Coronary Heart Disease Patients (ENRICHD) Study: The Effects of Treating Depression and Low Social Support on Clinical Events after Myocardial Infarction," *Journal of the American Medical Association* 289 (2003): 3106–16.

94. For more information on our study of mental health and mortality risk, see L. R. Martin, H. S. Friedman, J. S. Tucker, J. E. Schwartz, M. H. Criqui, D. L. Wingard, and C. Tomlinson-Keasey, "An Archival Prospective Study of Mental Health and Longevity," *Health Psychology* 14 (1995): 381–87.

95. More on the genetic study of depression is in A. Caspi, K. Sugden, T. E. Moffitt, A. Taylor, I. W. Craig, H. Harrington, J. McClay, J. Mill, J. Martin, A. Braithwaite, and R. Poulton, "Influences of Life Stress on Depression: Moderation by a Polymorphism in the 5-HTT Gene," *Science* 301, no. 5631 (2003): 386–89.

96. To read more about one of Vaillant's studies of the effects of World War II experiences, see K. A. Lee, G. E. Vaillant, W. C. Torrey, and G. H. Elder, "A 50-Year Prospective Study of the Psychological Sequelae of World War II Combat," *American Journal of Psychiatry* 152 (1995): 516–22.

97. For the study of Vietnam veterans, see A. C. Phillips, G. D. Batty,

C. R. Gale, I. J. Deary, D. Osborn, K. MacIntyre, and D. Carroll, "Generalized Anxiety Disorder, Major Depressive Disorder, and Their Comorbidity as Predictors of All-Cause and Cardiovascular Mortality: The Vietnam Experience Study," *Psychosomatic Medicine* 71 (2009): 395–403.

98. To read more about the Civil War veterans, see J. Pizarro, R. C. Silver, and J. Prause, "Physical and Mental Health Costs of Traumatic War Experiences among Civil War Veterans," *Archives of General Psychiatry* 63 (2006): 193–200.

99. For a study of finding meaning after the 9/11 terrorist attacks see J. A. Updegraff, R. C. Silver, and E. A. Holman, "Searching For and Finding Meaning In Collective Trauma: Results from a National Longitudinal Study of the 9/11 Terrorist Attacks," *Journal of Personality and Social Psychology* 95, no. 3 (2008): 709–22.

Chapter 15: Individual Paths to Health and Long Life

100. We have also met sons and daughters of people who *thought* they were Terman participants. But they were actually people who had been examined by Dr. Terman in some context but had never been admitted to the special group of 1,528 subjects. These contacts reminded us of all the mistakes and faulty inferences possible in complicated health research. We posted a reminder notice inside our lab door, near the Termanator sign, with our own investigative mantra: *Follow the Data!*

101. The National Institute on Aging funded much of our published empirical research. This book is an independent report of our interpretations and associated study, prepared on our own time; the findings herein are not intended to represent the views of the National Institute on Aging or any government agency.

Epilogue: Long Life and Public Health

102. To read more from the Rockefeller researchers, see J. P. Shonkoff, W. T. Boyce, and B. S. McEwen, "Neuroscience, Molecular Biology, and the Childhood Roots of Health Disparities: Building a New Framework for Health Promotion and Disease Prevention," *Journal of the American Medical Association* 301 (2009): 2252–59.

103. The Terman quote mentioning longevity comes from Terman and Oden, *Genetic Studies of Genius*, vol. 4, *The Gifted Child Grows Up*, 379.

· INDEX ·